The Sexual Teachings of the
JADE
DRAGON

Other Works by Hsi Lai

The Sexual Teachings of the White Tigress:
Secrets of the Female Taoist Masters

The Sexual Teachings

of the

JADE
DRAGON

Taoist Methods
for Male
Sexual
Revitalization

Hsi Lai

Destiny Books
Rochester, Vermont

Destiny Books
One Park Street
Rochester, Vermont 05767
www.InnerTraditions.com

Destiny Books is a division of Inner Traditions International

Library of Congress Cataloging-in-Publication Data
Lai, Hsi
The sexual teachings of the jade dragon : Taoists secrets for male
sexual revitalization / Hsi Lai.
p. cm.
Includes index
ISBN 0-89281-963-4
1. Sex instruction—Religious aspects—Taoism. 2. Sex—Religious
aspects—Taoism. I. Title: Taoists secrets for male sexual
revitalization. II. Title.
HQ64 .L259 2002
613.9'6—dc21
2002013383

Printed and bound in the United States

10 9 8 7 6 5 4 3 2 1

Text design by Virginia L. Scott Bowman
The book was typeset in Weiss with Weiss and Civet as display typefaces.

In every repose, a gourd of peach wine stands close to me.

With no aspirations of fame or greatness, I am truly content.

I am a True Man living among countless confused mortals; indeed it is so rare to meet a true immortal.

Are you willing to ride upon the azure dragon with me?

I will take you to where we all live in a wilderness by the open sea, atop a peak on the P'eng Lai islands.

We do not abstain from the pleasures and joys of life, just from the world's turmoil, which withers man's spirit into dust.

I can count the immortal dragons on my hands, so few there really are.

Do not listen to dictates of mortal men.

Leap upon this dragon and become a True Man.

—**White Tigress Manual**

Disclaimer

Because very few Asians actually have any knowledge of White Tigress practices, the reader should not judge the Asian culture as a whole or assume that any Asian person condones or believes in them. Most Asians will be hearing of these practices for the first time and will react to them as any other person would, with acceptance, disdain, or indifference.

The author and publisher disclaim any responsibility or liability for individuals who engage in any of the sexual practices described in this book. The materials presented here are meant to serve solely as a record and description of White Tigress ideology. Neither the author nor the publisher promotes any of the sexual methods or practices mentioned in this book, nor do they encourage any individual to engage in them.

It is the author's hope that anyone who would decide to undertake any of these practices, especially those requiring a sexual partner, would do so with great caution and consideration. None of the practices described in this book should be considered sexual amusements. Most of the practices described are very powerful psychologically and physiologically and therefore need to be approached carefully.

Note: The names of teachers and students of these teachings have been altered so as not to reveal their true identity or jeopardize their privacy.

Acknowledgments

Without the tenacious encouragement of Dr. Chen I would never have found myself in the beautiful world of the White Tigress nor would this book have ever become a reality. My deepest appreciation to him.

To Madame Lin, her daughter, and all the Tigresses under her tutelage. When I stayed in Taiwan to research this book all of them showed me so much kindness, provided me with so much support, and above all they so genuinely granted me all their trust. They changed my entire perception of not only sexual matters, but of women and love as well. I will forever be in their debt.

My deepest gratitude to all the Tigresses in America who helped answer so many questions, endured the hectic photography sessions, and wrote me so many clarifying letters. Their contributions were indispensable.

To everyone at Destiny Books who helped get this book into print. The enormous amount of time and effort given by the staff made this book so wonderful, so readable, and so beautiful.

I bow deeply to everyone with utmost gratitude and respect.

Contents

THREE

Revitalization of the Dragon Ching

57

FOUR
The Sexual Counsel of the Plain Girl
87

FIVE
Reverting Ching to the Brain
(The Yellow Stream or Stream of Life)
147

SIX
The Teachings of Taoist Master Yang Chu
167

SEVEN
The Bamboo Immortal
(The Jade Dragon Li Huang)
197

Afterword
234

About the Author
238

Index
239

Introduction

The Sexual Teachings of the Jade Dragon presents ancient Taoist methods for achieving male sexual revitalization and techniques of reverting sexual energy for heightened spiritual experiences and development. It provides both basic sexual methods for increasing sexual prowess and energy and for alleviating health concerns, as well as teaching methods for using this heightened sexual energy for the more subtle practices of achieving spiritual growth and immortality.

Even though consistent references are made specifically to the Taoist male roles of either the Jade Dragon or Green Dragon throughout the text, one is not required to be a traditional or bona fide Jade Dragon to apply any of the practices explained in this book. The information can be used by any male, as the majority of the material focuses on improving male sexual prowess and energy. This prowess and energy is, in part, what the ancient Taoists referred to as *ching*. In the broader sense, ching implies a person's entire physical and sexual constitution and function.

Within these unique Taoist sexual teachings, herein referred to as White Tigress teachings, there are two male roles. The first is called a Jade Dragon and the other a Green Dragon. A Jade Dragon is the traditional name of a male sexual partner that a White Tigress (female) might join with in her practice of these sexual-spiritual teachings. In addition to being her partner in these activities, he is also her benefactor and protector. A Jade Dragon and a White Tigress normally limit their practice time to three years, whereupon he returns to his more solitary Taoist practices, and she continues on with her practices with or without a Jade Dragon.

It can be said that a Jade Dragon is not a necessity for a White Tigress, although it is much easier for her to have a partner she totally trusts when engaging in the more transformational and spiritual techniques of this sexual practice. A Jade Dragon, however, is totally dependent upon acquiring a White Tigress, for without her he could never develop his sexual energy to the level needed for experiencing the spiritual heights to which he aspires.

Aside from being her copracticer, benefactor, and protector he also plays the role of being the voyeur, while the Tigress is the exhibitionist. Within his voyeuristic role, a practice called Gazing at the Green Dragons, he stimulates his sexual energy to very intense mental states so that he may experience the inner alchemical experience of The Yellow Stream, which is induced by driving the *qi* energy up along the spine into the brain, and thus ensuring his development towards longevity and immortality.

A Green Dragon is a sexual partner or surrogate lover of a White Tigress, used by her purely for the purposes of acquiring his sexual energy and semen. Unlike a Jade Dragon, Green Dragons are indispensable and crucial to a White Tigress's practice and progress, for even if she had a Jade Dragon he would be unable to provide her with the necessary sexual energy and semen needed over the three-year practice period. Encounters with Green Dragons are very disciplined sexual affairs, and a great deal of preparation and emphasis is put on finding and meeting them. In some cases a Green Dragon is made aware of his role and in some cases is totally unaware of it, based on the sole discretion of the White Tigress.

A Jade Dragon engages in the sexual practices described in this book for three years in order to develop and intensify his sexual energy, his ching. After the three-year period, he will most likely seek to partake in the more male-focused practices such as those explained in chapter 4, The Sexual Counsel of the Plain Girl, or simply practice Taoist self-cultivation methods of inner alchemy and meditation.

In almost all spiritual traditions there appear frequent references to those who achieved spiritual enlightenment in nine years of practice. We see this, for example, in Bodhidharma's nine years of wall gazing and in the Taoists Chang San Feng's and Lu Tung Pin's nine years of refining the elixir of immortality. The Jade Dragon too looks at his career of achieving immortality within nine years, three of which he spends with a White Tigress. White Tigresses themselves practice for nine years. But to the Jade Dragon the first three years of practicing with a White Tigress are the most important, for they lay the foundation for fully developing *ching*, the first of three major energies to be developed—the other two being *qi* and *shen*, breath and spirit.

The information provided in this book comes from a text entitled *White Tigress Manual*, compiled in 1748 by the then matriarch of the White Tigress sect, Chin Hua. In 1986 I first met with the present-day matriarch of the White Tigress sect, a Madame Lin, in Taiwan. With her help I began compiling and translating various materials from the manual, which have resulted so far in two volumes—*The Sexual Teachings of the White Tigress* and this book, *The Sexual Teachings of the Jade Dragon*.

The purpose of *The Sexual Teachings of the White Tigress* was primarily to explain the practices and philosophy of the White Tigress, a female who has undertaken disciplined sexual and spiritual practices in order to attain the condition of a Taoist immortaless. The roles and specific practices of the Tigress's male counterpart, the Jade Dragon, were only briefly described in that volume. In *The Sexual Teachings of the Jade Dragon* I focus primarily on the practices and philosophy of the Jade Dragon. Though this book details techniques for male sexual revitalization, I recommend that men read *The Sexual Teachings of the White Tigress* as well, especially those who are inclined to take on the more traditional practice of forming the White Tigress–Jade Dragon union for sexual-spiritual cultivation.

The methods and information provided in this book were originally transmitted to men from a female White Tigress. The Tigress's goal was to have men around her who could provide her with greater sexual energy and more potent amounts of semen for her sexual-spiritual restoration practices—Congealing the Dragon's Jade and Absorbing the Dragon's Breath. These practices serve as the precursors for her achieving physical restoration and spiritual illumination and for forming her spirit immortaless fetus. Thus she embarks upon her final quest of becoming an Immortaless. She would transmit these teachings to her Jade Dragon, provided she had one, and, if she chose, to her favored Green Dragons (sexual surrogates).

As in all Taoist self-cultivation practices for achieving immortality, the three energies—or Three Treasures—of ching (sexual and physical energy), qi (vital and breath energy), and shen (mental and spiritual energy) must be restored and refined to their optimum condition. The main difference in these practices is whether the male

Taoist chooses to use celibacy or sexual activity in refining the ching energy. Both celibate and sexual methods have their pros and cons. Celibacy can efficiently restore a man's ching but can also cause various health problems and in some cases cause the mental distress associated with fanaticism, thus hurting the shen. Sexual activity can more expediently refine the ching but can cause physical and mental problems associated with sexual overindulgence. However, with the unquestionable reality that sexual energy is the most powerful of all human energies, the use of sexual techniques is the most expedient and efficient manner in which to revitalize and develop these Three Treasures.

The practices of the Jade Dragon make use of a balanced interchange of brief periods of celibacy, revitalization of sexual energy and functions, sexual activity without ejaculation, sexual activity with ejaculation, voyeurism, and internal energy work with the Three Treasures (normally called Taoist alchemy or forming the Elixir of Immortality). The strengthening of the ching through these practices is paramount to the production of qi and the development of the shen. So in the end, a male seeking optimum health and immortality can follow either the celibate or the sexual path, keeping in mind that the two most harmful missteps are sexual overindulgence and sexual denial. Both dissipate the ching at an accelerated rate and thus shorten a man's life span, as both over-and underindulgence damage physical and mental health.

An Overview of the Chapters

The first chapter of this book, *Leaping Over the Dragon Gate*, outlines the purpose, practices, and goals of a Jade Dragon and also includes advice for Green Dragons in relation to the interaction with a White Tigress. Since the particulars concerning the Jade and Green Dragons were just lightly touched upon in *The Sexual Teachings of the White Tigress*, their roles are made much clearer here.

The second chapter provides the correlations of the Eight Diagrams *(pa kua)* of the I Ching (Book of Changes) with the eight basic types of Jade Stems (penises), and the Five Element *(wu hsing)* correspondences of the five basic types of the glans penis and the five types of semen quality.

The philosophies and correlations behind the Eight Diagrams and Five Elements are integral to everything in Chinese physiology and philosophy. In fact, the Chinese believe that unless these correlations between the physical and philosophical exist, the subject at hand will have little worth or applicability. Therefore, it was no surprise to find in the *White Tigress Manual* these types of correlations, the purpose being to reveal to both a White Tigress and a Jade Dragon the positive or negative functions of the male's sexual reproductive system, which is extremely important for determining the maintenance or revitalization necessary for optimal sexual partner.

Chapter 3 discusses various methods of revitalization of male sexual energy, including herbal remedies and specialized exercises for developing heightened sexual energy, enlarging the penis, increasing semen quality and quantity, and cures for specific sexual dysfunctions. This chapter is about revitalizing and maintaining a strong level of ching (sexual energy and prowess) in the male. This chapter is the crux of the entire book, as it provides the male with self-sexual empowerment methods that will help him develop his ching to optimal levels, thus making him a prime candidate for becoming a Jade or Green Dragon for the White Tigress.

Chapter 4 is the White Tigress version of the ancient sex manual called *The Sexual Counsel of the Plain Girl Classic (Su Nu Ching)*. It covers a wide range of sexual techniques and therapies for the male and even some for the female. The material of this classic text falls into the category of Dual Sexual Cultivation, which in practice has more benefit for the male than the female. Hence, the White Tigress views these practices more as a curative process for her Jade Dragon, but not as a standard or continual practice, as they deal mostly with sexual intercourse. Since her main goal is to keep her Jade Dragon physically, mentally, and sexually healthy, these age-old techniques and advice prove very useful within the White Tigress and Jade Dragon practices.

Chapter 5 covers the deeper alchemical practices of Opening the Original Cavity in the brain and Reverting Ching to the Brain (illumination of the mind). These are integral conjunctive processes needed for experiencing the effects of the spiritual state called the Yellow Stream, the achievement for both illumination and for creating the immortal spiritual fetus. This is achieved through four activities: meditative processes, conducive sexual postures, breathing techniques, and using sexual energy during voyeuristic experiences. It should also be noted that any of these four practices can be applied separately or in conjunction with one another, as each method is designed to provide the mental intensity and physical means by which to cause the sexual energy and qi to rise upward along the spine to create the illumination experience. The Jade Dragon, however, wanting to ensure his accomplishment of the Yellow Stream, applies all four methods simultaneously.

Chapter 6 comes from the Han dynasty Taoist work called *The Book of Lieh Tzu*. The seventh chapter of that work, entitled Yang Chu, is presented here. Many scholars have questioned why Lieh Tzu included a record of Yang Chu's philosophy, considering that when taken at face value it seems hedonistic and egotistical, with its stated views appearing almost completely contrary to the views expressed in the other chapters in the Lieh Tzu. But if read as an exercise in using extremism against the extremist Confucian views of his day, the work is actually more Taoistic in tone than most other Taoist writings.

The *White Tigress Manual* includes this Yang Chu chapter of the *Lieh Tzu* as its first section, which is about the deportments of a Jade Dragon, because it deems the Jade Dragon philosophy to be an undercurrent for all true Taoist thinking. In light of this, Yang Chu goes out of his way to denounce the pretense of reputation, conformity, and morality, taking issue with any conventions that hinder the individual from acting freely on his natural instincts and living life to the fullest, without interference from those who preach doctrines that attempt to change a person's right to follow his own *tao* (way).

Yang Chu provides a philosophical backdrop for both the Jade Dragon and the White Tigress; no matter what age we live in, the current moral issues attempt to gather people into one common frame of thinking, whether religious or civil. Yang Chu, however, stresses complete individualism and non-conformity, advocating that all people live and think in complete indifference to the thoughts and dictates of others who seek to change and convert them into their way of thinking and behaviors.

Chapter 7 is a brief biography of the Taoist Li Huang (1712 – ?), who went by his initiate name of Bamboo Immortal. For three years Li Huang studied under the White Tigress matriarch Chin Hua as a Jade Dragon with her disciple Ling I. His personal record reveals some of his early influences which led him to Taoism and to the practices of the Jade Dragon, and then finally to the life of a hermit. His story is a valuable and rare work that outlines in a personal admission the benefits he derived from being a Jade Dragon. Written in a typically polite Taoist manner, Li Huang's narrative provides numerous insights into the role and practices of the Jade Dragon.

Definition of Terms

The following terms appear frequently in the text, and brief explanations of them are provided here in order to prevent any confusion.

White Tigress. A female who has undertaken disciplined sexual and spiritual practices of acquiring male essence, specifically sexual energy, in order to realize her full feminine potential and the condition of an Immortaless. Over time the various practices of these women eventually led to the development and formation of the White Tigress societies. Though they were never established as an organized school, White Tigress lineages were passed down in secret to certain women—and men—who rejected the views of the moralists and Confucians, the predominant creators of social norms.

Taoism. The first indigenous philosophy of China. Taoism, at its heart, presents a philosophy of living naturally within the world, a doctrine of noncontention and noninterference with the world—Taoists were the original freethinkers in Chinese society. Taoist philosophy is primarily based on the work of the Yellow Emperor (Huang Ti, the attributed author of the *Internal Medicine Classic*), Lao Tzu and his work the *Tao Te Ching*, Chuang Tzu's writings in the *Chuang Tzu*, and Ko Hung's *Pao P'u Tzu*. These writings and teachings experienced a great deal of interpretation throughout China's history, and so Taoism has been divided into many sects, schools, and divergent practices.

These divisions were also created because Taoist classical writings can be and were interpreted and practiced in any of the three following manners: as internal alchemy (the processes for forming the elixir of immortality), as contemplative philosophy (the methods of achieving tranquillity and the Tao), and as hygiene practices (physical restoration methods). (Certain sects of Taoism also have a very deep history and involvement with ritual-magic practices, but not within the teachings presented here.) The more traditional Taoist schools recognized and adapted all three interpretations simultaneously and did not discard one in favor of another. The White Tigress adheres to all three as well, first undergoing the sexual regeneration, then the spiritual alchemy, and lastly the contemplative philosophy—blending and developing all three over a nine-year period.

Sexually speaking, the Taoists viewed men and women as equal partners in the interplay of creating supreme harmony and immortality—just as Heaven and Earth and yin and yang forces of nature must balance each other to achieve fulfillment and harmony. So too men and women can balance each other and create a supreme harmony of their spiritual energies. In the *White Tigress Manual* it states, "Look to what created you to discover what will restore and immortalize you." Sexual energy brought you into this world and likewise can provide the means of providing perfect health and longevity.

Immortality. A wide divergence of meaning is given to the concept of immortality in the many schools of Taoism. Some schools believe in actual physical immortality, wherein the body can be preserved as long as a person deems necessary. Another meaning is that the spirit and consciousness remain intact and lucid during death and so would be able to direct the self to immortal paradises or heavenly realms of existence rather than its returning to this earthly realm. The most practical meaning is that the person lives beyond one hundred years in good health or as the Chinese say, "retaining youthfulness within old age." To the Jade Dragon and White Tigress, however, immortality carries the ideas of living with optimum health, living longer while maintaining a youthful physical appearance and disposition, and achieving lucid consciousness upon death.

Restoring youthfulness. The object of restoring youthfulness is to recapture the physical condition of the adolescent years, not to revert back to the original height of a fourteen-year-old. Rather, the skin, hair, penis, vagina, breasts, muscle tone, hearing, and eyesight will all feel and function pretty much as they did during late adolescence and early adulthood. Some of the physical sensations and energy of the adolescent years are also reexperienced. The Jade Dragon believes that a man can become five to fifteen years younger, depending on the age at which he begins practicing and how much aging damage has occurred. As a Taoist proverb says, "No one can cheat death and old age, but death can certainly be impeded and life can be prolonged."

Qi. "Energy," "breath," and "vital force" are all interpretations of qi. In brief, it is the internal vital energy that is stimulated in acupuncture, and qi is the energy that animates all life forms. The very warmth of the human body is a result of qi, which is thought to be like an inherent oxygen in the body and blood that stimulates vitality and stamina. In Chinese thinking the body can live for a certain period of time without food, breath, or blood circulation. But without qi it cannot exist for even a moment.

Ching. The very primal urge people have to reproduce themselves, the behavior we apply in expressing sexual desire, the substances contained within sexual fluids—the regenerative force—are all ching, or sexual energy.

The orgasm is the most intense human experience. No other experience is as totally focused or concentrated, providing not only a great sense of pleasure, release, and relaxation but also a powerful enhancement of all the senses. Of all the forces within human beings, sexual energy is the strongest, and it is expressed in our daily life in countless ways—from consumption of food to sexual activity.

The orgasm emits sexual energy from the body, not only in fluids, but also as a substantive psychological force. The Jade Dragon learns to revert the energy of his orgasm back into his body for both physical and spiritual purposes. The White Tigress discovers how to absorb and make full use of the fluids and energies of her own orgasm as well as the male's orgasm to benefit her spiritual and physiological progress. We in the West have yet to fully comprehend the intrinsic connection between sexuality and spirituality. To the Taoist the sexual and spiritual refinement of *ching* (sexual energy, physical functions), *qi* (vital energy, breath), and *shen* (spirit, consciousness)—the Three Treasures—is the secret with which to unlock not only the restoration of our youthfulness but our immortality as well.

Sexual energy, if directed in a negative manner, can cause numerous ailments from eating disorders to psychological traumas. Sex, no matter your preference, whether you desire it or abstain from it, is still the undercurrent of both your physical condition and your psychological temperament. Each human being has the choice to use it either positively or negatively.

Concluding Remarks

Taoism can be seen as three primary practices: an internal alchemical practice, a contemplative philosophical practice, and a hygiene practice. All Taoist methods fall under one of these three categories, and in some schools, all three are propagated and practiced simultaneously. The teachings in this book fall under the category of alchemical practices, with the goals of achieving health, longevity, and immortality.

There is so much more to these sexual teachings than just developing greater sexual prowess and sharing sexual intimacy with a White Tigress. In the end, it is the melding of sexual and spiritual energy that provides the Jade Dragon and White Tigress with the benefits of health, longevity, and wisdom.

The first topic covered here is for strengthening the penis, increasing semen quantity and quality, and developing sexual energy. Taoism asserts that the ching and qi are developed in the lower abdomen but expressed through the penis and breath. The shen (spirit) is developed in the brain and expressed through the eyes. This work focuses on those developments to create the means by which any man can progress in either or both of his energies, sexual and spiritual.

For men who wish to be either a Jade or Green Dragon within the White Tigress practice it is important to begin by first strengthening and developing all aspects of the ching. These results are achieved through the use of specific herbs and exercises developed by Taoists centuries ago. A White Tigress needs to find men who can provide these aspects of ching. Every man, whether a practicing Taoist or not, seeks to maintain high sexual energy and prowess.

There is a lot of information in this book, and I hope it is all put to good use. I now offer a piece of advice that I discovered in my own practice: Enlarging the penis and enhancing sexual prowess should also mean enlarging your perception of sexuality and your understanding and appreciation of women. Treat your partners well, be kind and gentle, and allow them to benefit from your revitalized sexual energy.

ONE

Leaping over the Dragon Gate

龍
門

> *The barrier between mortality and immortality is the Dragon Gate.*
> *With great effort it must be leapt over, like a fish hurling itself from the safety of the water.*
> *The real struggle lies within the self; conformity and laxness are what prevent you from leaping to the other side of the Dragon Gate.*
>
> **—White Tigress Manual**

Jade Dragons

The term *Jade Dragon* is a euphemism for both the penis and the partner of a Tigress. In these practices he is the one with whom she practices, for whom she performs, in whom she confides, and on whom she depends for protection, support, and discipline. The Jade Dragon engages in these sexual practices with a Tigress for the following important reasons:

- Through the voyeuristic practice called Gazing at the Green Dragon (see page 24), a Jade Dragon can build his sexual energy to the levels that will ensure full potency, providing the heightened stimulation of his ching for inducing the experience of the Yellow Stream. This practice will also cause him to empathize with, understand, and be more sensitive toward the female so as to draw out his yin aspects much more readily and fully.

- To revitalize his ching (semen and sexual energy) through specific sexually oriented exercises and herbal regimens, so that he can regain his health and youthfulness and render his internal energies (ching and qi) strong enough to aid in stimulating the Yellow Stream.

- The Transformational Techniques—the methods of Opening the Original Cavity and Reverting Ching to the Brain—and specific sexual postures will help ensure his ability to complete the Yellow Stream and will provide him with accentuated health and longevity.

- Beyond all these disciplined practices, exercises, and regimens the Jade Dragon gains a new perspective, emotionally and philosophically, about himself, life, sexuality, spirituality, and women. In Taoist philosophy it is said that the Dragon (male) and Tigress (female) are trapped in eternal battle with each other. Harmony is achieved only when each individual blends with and creates illumination in the other. The roles played during the deportments of the Jade Dragon and White Tigress are designed specifically to ensure this blending.

The mineral jade has long been considered by the Chinese as the semen of dragons or "Dragon Jade." According to legend

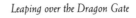

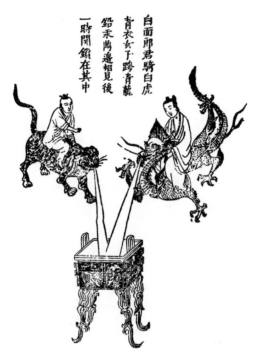

龍虎交媾圖

白面郎君騎白虎
青衣女下跨青龍
鉛汞嘔逽相見後
一時閉鎖在其中

To whiten the face the boy bestrides
the White Tigress.
The green-robed girl sits astride the
Green Dragon.
The power of the lead and mercury
fuse in the cauldron, at once the
gate is locked from within.

A Diagram of the Dragon and Tiger Refining Their Essences

dragons, like some fish, do not ejaculate inside their female counterparts but on them, and the females are impregnated by absorption through their gills or scales. Dragon semen that is not absorbed falls to the earth and congeals as precious jade, which acts as a restorative element.

To the Chinese, dark green jade, the most precious of all, is symbolic of longevity. To a female, who is a representation of earth, the semen of the dragon (male) should be congealed on her to produce the jadelike elixir of health and longevity. Hence, in connection with the explanation of White Tigress and Green Dragon, the Dragon (penis) deposits semen (white) onto the face of the Tigress (female). When the semen congeals it becomes the essence for restoring youthfulness (jade).

Being a Jade Dragon

The Jade Dragon's role in the White Tigress's practices is without question extremely difficult. Just as few women can actually become full-fledged White Tigresses, very few men can actually be practicing Jade Dragons. The reason for this is because the male must be void of jealously, attachment, and lack of discipline while also maintaining an intense sexual-spiritual relationship with the White Tigress. Indeed the majority of men would most likely find the reconciliation of intense sexual practices with simultaneous disciplined spiritual practices beyond their scope of acceptance and capability. Without being deeply disciplined within Taoism it is highly improbable that any male could be successful in this role. But those males who do have the background and discipline will find this role vastly rewarding on both a physical and spiritual level.

A White Tigress seeks a Jade Dragon to secure herself a practice partner and physical protector, financial security, and emotional support. For three years he is considered her lover and benefactor, and she does nothing sexually without his knowledge. He in turn needs to be assured of her total commitment and affection during the practice period and has to be certain that she will never use the practice as a means of attaining wealth or material possessions. In repayment for what he gives her and her ability to practice, she provides him not only with a perfect mistress relationship but also with the means to restore his own youthfulness and begin his cultivation of immortality.

The relationship of a Jade Dragon and a White Tigress is based on a sexual practice, and as in many relationships, money and love are intrinsically connected. The Jade Dragon has to be able to meet the financial demands of the relationship during the period of practice. The White Tigress must never take advantage of his role as the financial provider and never ask for anything beyond the agreed-upon conditions. If money issues are taken care of from the beginning, the Dragon and Tigress can both practice more easily and comfortably.

The Jade Dragon and White Tigress normally live separately, even if in the same house, where she has her own room for sleeping. One night per week she enters the Jade Dragon's bedroom and requests to sleep next to him for the whole night. If they both agree, the White Tigress could use this opportunity to have intercourse with him. On no other occasions do they ever sleep in the same bed, unless they are traveling together. When this is the case, she sleeps with him each night. When they return home, they resume their usual sleeping arrangements.

Traditionally, a White Tigress stayed with her Jade Dragon during the three-year practice period and then continued on without him. Others, however, would choose to secure a new Jade Dragon or stay with the same one for another three-year period.

For the Jade Dragon, the White Tigress practices are like a curtain that is drawn open to let him see women, sex, and himself from a completely different and transcendental perspective. When the Jade Dragon engages in secretly watching his White Tigress with Green Dragons, he can achieve very intense states of sexual stimulation, which, through visualization and breathing techniques, can then be used as a catalyst to induce his ching and qi up his spine and into his brain. As will be seen in this book, Jade Dragon practices rely on three primary means in which to induce the ching and qi up the spine. The first is contained in the methods of retention and reverting of his orgasm when engaged in sexual activity with his White Tigress; the second is using voyeurism to provide intense sexual stimulation; and the third is making use of all the methods for revitalizing his ching.

To some it may seem odd that a Jade Dragon would go through all these disciplined regimes to increase his sexual prowess and energy and then not use those improvements for his own sexual satisfaction. Yet the Jade Dragon has a much higher and more spiritual purpose. Sexuality is but a stepping stone for him. In the end, his revitalization of sexual energy, his retention of and reverting semen ejaculation, and his inducing intense sexual stimulation with voyeurism is akin to storing and accumulating energy so that it may be directed and focused to provide the catalyst for experiencing an event greater than just the experience of orgasm, namely the Yellow Stream (see chapter 5).

The constant dissipation of semen leads only to old age, sickness, and death. A man's ching is the basis of his physical health, and to haphazardly and frequently dissipate it is to throw his health away. The preservation of ching can provide greater health and heightened spiritual experiences. Even though it is said that ejaculation is to be preserved, it doesn't mean a man never ejaculates, as that would make him celibate. Biologically men need to experience orgasm from time to time, but even this needs to be disciplined in accordance with the age of the man (see chapter 4). It is also true that Jade Dragons, because of their heightened sexual energy and voyeurism, will find it difficult not to ejaculate on occasion. The goal is not to prevent all ejaculation but to learn how to control it. This is the crux of the Jade Dragon practices, for with increased sexual prowess must come increased sexual discipline.

Traditionally, after a three-year practice period ended, a Jade Dragon would go into seclusion to meditate and refine his essences for longevity and immortality. At this time he would either drop sexual activity altogether or remain with his wife and concubines to enjoy this newfound sexual vitality and youthfulness. Some Jade Dragons also became teachers who trained White Tigresses.

The Taoist ideal for a man has always been for him to join a hermitage or monastery and begin his meditation and alchemy practice while still an adolescent; thus he would never have to go through any sexual restoration practices. However, most males are not fortunate enough to undertake spiritual practices in adolescence. Their sexual energy from going through puberty is then too destructive for meditation practices, and they have to wait until such time as they are stable and calm enough to learn meditation.

There are two unbreakable rules for a Jade Dragon. The first is that he must have sex only with the White Tigress during the practice period. If he secretly or openly has sex with another woman without the White Tigress's permission, she can end the agreement, take the money set aside for her, keep the gifts and other property, and leave. If that is the Jade Dragon's character, then he isn't serious about the practice or about her. Such actions would negate the benefits they had both received from the practice and would also be very damaging to them psychologically; for once a White Tigress can no longer trust her Jade Dragon, there is really no use for him, and keeping him would only cause her harm. This rule, however, is not a traditional one. In earlier times fidelity was not required because men could maintain a wife and concubines. The rule of fidelity was obviously inserted into the practices within the last one hundred years or so.

The second unbreakable rule is that no physical violence can be directed at the White Tigress. This practice is a form of the anti-abuse and harassment laws we see today. A Jade Dragon who physically harms a White Tigress suffers greatly for his misdeed. The punishment, clearly stated to the Jade Dragon candidate, is instituted by the White Tigress's teacher, who can hire thugs to administer a severe beating. Depending on the severity of the abuse, the Jade Dragon can be rendered a eunuch. Presently the punishments for Jade Dragon abuses are not as severe as they were in former times and are more or less just simple cases of being dismissed from her life and practices.

Other rules include: the Jade Dragon cannot force a White Tigress into prostitution, cannot not force a White Tigress to have intercourse if she chooses not to, and cannot end their agreement for any other reason than her having broken the rules. Because of the stringency of these rules in the past the records show very few reports of any abuses. Madame Lin thought the main reason for this was that men who were interested in becoming Jade Dragons were usually more interested in Taoist alchemical disciplines than just sex. Therefore, the "breed" of these men was of a much gentler persuasion than what a sing-song girl (prostitute) would attract.

No man should ever take on the responsibility or honor of being a Jade Dragon without total commitment to the White Tigress. How they decide to lead their lives after completing the practice period is up to them, but during the practice period, the Jade Dragon must be completely loyal to, encouraging, and supportive of the White Tigress.

A Jade Dragon who successfully completes a three-year practice period with a White Tigress is considered to be qualified to instruct White Tigresses. If the White Tigress recommends him to her teacher and the Jade Dragon makes a financial contribution to both the White Tigress and her teacher for that privilege, he can then receive further teachings and is allowed to begin his own lineage. When a Jade Dragon becomes a teacher he is called a White Tiger.

The Jade Dragon and White Tigress do not engage in the more popular Taoist practices of Dual Sexual Cultivation, even though some of the Transformational Techniques are quite similar. Dual Sexual Cultivation methods are primarily for the male, and although they provide some aspects of restoration for the female, they are not nearly as effective or focused as the restorative benefits of the White Tigress practices. Despite this, the Jade Dragon will on occasion, especially before or after the Tigress's first three-year restoration period, engage in Dual Sexual Cultivation practices in order to cure or prevent various mental and physical illnesses or deficiencies. Hence, because the majority of male readers will not become traditional Jade Dragons, the methods of Dual Sexual Cultivation are included in this work (see chapter 4), making the book more valuable to all male readers.

Gazing at the Green Dragon

The basis of Gazing at the Green Dragon was discussed briefly in *The Sexual Teachings of the White Tigress*, but since that book focused primarily on methods for women, the male role will be more fully explained here. This practice makes use of external physical visualization (voyeurism). The primary technique for Gazing at the Green Dragon is the act of actually watching a White Tigress perform sexual acts with a Green Dragon, either openly or secretly. The idea is to create intense sexual stimulation of the Jade Dragon to both strengthen his ching (sexual energy) and to act as a catalyst for initiating the process of Reverting Ching to the Brain (see chapter 5).

How a White Tigress and Jade Dragon decide to accomplish his watching her with a Green Dragon is purely at their discretion. Depending on what makes the Jade Dragon most comfortable, he decides whether to watch with or without the Green Dragon's knowledge. It can also be the case that certain Green Dragons feel too intimidated if they know they are being watched, while some would be quite comfortable. The Jade Dragon takes this information into account as well. Whatever method they use, it is important for the Jade Dragon to witness her activities clearly and without disturbance.

It is not absolutely necessary that a Jade Dragon watch his Tigress with a Green Dragon—although it can be helpful to both of them. He should, however, always try to be in a nearby room or within earshot of her, if for no other reason than to help her feel protected, allowing her to indulge herself to the fullest extent with the Green Dragon.

Some Jade Dragons, on the other hand, prefer to simply hear about the White Tigress's encounters when they are alone together. But whether a Jade Dragon watches her encounter, wants to hear about it, or does not want to know is purely up to him. A White Tigress always honors his request concerning this aspect of their relationship. It is also important that he not participate in the sexual activity, as his purpose is to watch or listen and use the stimulation for developing his ching.

When watching the White Tigress with a Green Dragon, the Jade Dragon should be seated in a comfortable position, preferably in a seated meditation posture. Holding the base of his penis tightly with his left hand so as to trap the blood within the penis shaft, he applies muscular contractions to the glans penis, doing so thirty-six times slowly and in succession, while intently watching the White Tigress perform with the Green Dragon.

Next he takes his thumb and index finger of the left hand and places them tightly around the base of the penis, maintaining pressure. Then with the right hand, again using his thumb and index finger, he makes thirty-six consecutive tight, rhythmic squeezing movements directly beneath the glans penis. Keeping the pressure of the left hand upon the base of the penis, he again performs another thirty-six muscular contractions of the glans penis.

When these two techniques have been completed he repeatedly performs Dragon Twists Pillar, as presented in the Nine Jade Dragon Exercises (see page 71), until he feels that his erection is completely full and he senses a slight pain or aching in the groin and pubic area. At this point he closes his eyes and performs Reverting the Energy of Erections (see chapter 5), so that he may retain the energy internally and so that he can calm the intensity.

If at any point in his gazing the Jade Dragon senses that he is about to ejaculate, he should tighten his grip around the bottom of the penis shaft with his left and apply a firm pinching to the tip of the penis with his right thumb and index finger. (See Preventing Premature Ejaculations in chapter 3). He should then visualize the sexual energy reverting back into the kidney region, rolling his eyes upward as if gazing at the innermost portion of the top of his head (the *Pai Hui* cavity), draw up the anal muscle, place the tongue on the roof of his mouth, and breathe in deeply, holding the breath until the sensation subsides. If ejaculation occurs he should not engage himself with the White Tigress sexually but should privately practice Opening the Original Cavity.

After Gazing at the Green Dragon is over, the Jade Dragon should either engage the White Tigress in one of the three techniques of Sexual Positions for Inducing the Yellow Stream or he should practice the method for Opening the Original Cavity by himself (see chapter 5). It is extremely important for the Jade Dragon to discipline himself to do one or both of these after having watched the White Tigress with a Green Dragon. This is for two reasons: first, the Jade Dragon develops the discipline of internalizing the energy built up from the voyeurism, and second, he does not dissipate that energy and his ejaculation solely out of lust. It is extremely important that he makes use of his heightened sexual energy so that it is internalized, thus not only accentuating his Three Treasures but also becoming a driving force for the experience of the Yellow Stream.

During all of the previous activities the breath should be kept low in the abdomen; even when holding the breath it should feel as though it is retained in the *tan t'ien* (literally "the field of the elixir," a point in the lower abdomen where qi will accumulate and develop). If the breathing becomes labored or rapid, the Jade Dragon should close his eyes, release his hands from the penis, and focus on calming the breath. When the breath feels normal and low again, he may resume the practice.

Beyond being just an exercise in voyeurism, Gazing at the Green Dragon is meant to aid the Jade Dragon's ability to accumulate a high degree of ching, which is akin to adding more fuel to fire so the melting process of refining raw iron ore into steel can occur. This is an analogy often used by Taoists when speaking of cultivating internal energy. The greater the ching, the greater the qi, and the greater the impact on the shen.

It is very important for the Jade Dragon to interact with the White Tigress in the most supportive and encouraging manner possible during all the practices, and this is especially true for the practices that include Green Dragons. Not only must the Jade Dragon assist her in her daily self-practices, but he must also assist her in her quest for finding suitable Green Dragons. The following list is an overview of how a Jade Dragon should conduct himself concerning the White Tigress's practice of finding and practicing with Green Dragons:

- The first and most important matter is to discuss at length the method(s) the White Tigress will use to find suitable Green Dragons, and what part, if any, the Jade Dragon should play in helping her secure them. For example, if she chooses to do massage, then it will be the Jade Dragon's responsibility to help with locating and creating the environment in which she can do this. It is extremely important that his role in these matters be clearly defined so that neither person feels that they have too much or too little involvement.

- Next they must clearly define the means by which the Jade Dragon will or will not take part in the practice of Gazing at the Green Dragon. This will help determine how the White Tigress secures Green Dragons and under what conditions she has encounters with them, thus making this a discipline within itself. For example, if she chooses to perform massage and will not seek Green Dragons outside of her business, he would be able discern his ability and manner in which to watch her.

- Finally, they must discuss and decide how they will or will not engage with each other after she is finished with the Green Dragon. That is, will they practice one of the three Sexual Positions for Inducing the Yellow Stream, or will he go off by himself to practice Opening the Original Cavity? Or will they alternate methods or perhaps do both? There is no standard for this, and the decisions depend on all the varying factors of the methods she uses and their emotional comfort levels.

The Jade Dragon must be very careful not to demand that the White Tigress perform in a certain way and he must not interfere with how she acquires Green Dragons. He must be able to sit back and be of help when asked, yet indifferent when not asked, allowing her the comfort and space to act in the manner in which she is most comfortable and confident. If he feels she has made errors he should not scold or give harsh criticism, but should inform her in a calm, suggestive manner. The underlying goal should always be to create harmony. For the Jade Dragon, all the practices in which he engages should be regulated with an intention of creating tranquillity and relaxation in both the White Tigress and himself.

Green Dragons

Women are flowers, the very essence of a man's desires and enjoyment. Be kind and respectful, and she will return it with granting her favors. Be thoughtful and generous, and she will grant your deepest desires. Be loving, and she will love back. Above all, whether seeking her return or the first interlude, patient perseverance will always win her favors in the end.

—White Tigress Manual

A Green Dragon serves no other purpose than to be a provider of semen and sexual energy, and he does so in most cases unknowingly. A Green Dragon is led to believe that he is being seduced by the White Tigress purely for sexual pleasure.

These men are called Green Dragons for two reasons. In earlier Chinese history the color green represented the hue of a new sprouting plant, and this was associated with ching and youthfulness. After a White Tigress had sexual interplay with a Green Dragon and she depleted him of all his sexual essences and energy, he would be symbolically considered a "fallen dragon." This is taken from an allusion in the I Ching: "A fallen dragon withering away upon the earth." The penis is associated symbolically with the dragon, and the female symbolizes the earth. The image of a flaccid penis, drained of sexual energy by a female, was figuratively seen as a dragon lying down and withering upon the earth.

The other symbolic meaning of a Green Dragon is that of green reptiles: snakes, lizards, crocodiles, and so on. Chinese medicine has for centuries considered the oils from these animals highly effective in treating skin imperfections and diseases as well as curing blood disorders. Green "dragons" were considered the earthly species of heavenly dragons and so could provide numerous health benefits to human beings.

The ideal Green Dragon was a man who ejaculated a large quantity of thick, white semen. Semen that had a grayish color was avoided because it meant the Green Dragon was suffering from some illness. Semen that was clear was also avoided because it indicated that the male was an alcoholic or masturbated too frequently, thus he was only able to ejaculate seminal fluid.

Semen that contains a hint of red is normal. Men can sometimes have some blood in their semen, but this happens very infrequently. The Chinese say it is a sign of the feminine aspect in all males—just as females can produce a whitish, semenlike sexual secretion, which is a minor sign of the masculine aspect.

The Green Dragon is in every sense like a drone to a queen bee. In the traditional practices, a Green Dragon was not released until he had a minimum of three consecutive orgasms in a single encounter, and the White Tigress would fellate him daily until all his strength was depleted and he could take no more—so hurried and fanatical were some White Tigresses. Modern-day White Tigresses follow practices that have been modified in some ways, but the essential elements of the tradition remain.

Being a Green Dragon

There is no other way to become a Green Dragon than to be selected by a White Tigress. Even though most Green Dragons are completely unaware of being the subject of a White Tigress's practice, there are still several rules and requirements placed upon the Green Dragon, most of which is left unspoken.

- The White Tigress only seeks men who are polite, clean, and toward whom she has good feelings.
- Since the main method and purpose of her practice with Green Dragons is the performance of oral sex, she seeks men who both enjoy it and do not demand other sexual activity. She may request other types of activity, however.
- She limits her encounters with any particular man to nine separate times, so as not to create too much attachment between them. Within each of these nine encounters she will bring him to orgasm no more than three times, but only if he is capable of this. In earlier times it appears that a Green Dragon was not released from her seductions until he was completely spent and could no longer achieve erection or orgasm, but this practice has been relaxed in present times.

    After the nine encounters she allows at least one six-week

period before beginning another nine encounters with him—mostly because if she keeps seeing him too frequently the sexual intensity will diminish.

- Even though it is entirely up to the discretion of the White Tigress as to her method of procuring Green Dragons—for example, some do massage, others prefer clandestine meetings, some prefer datelike encounters—no White Tigress spends an entire night with a Green Dragon. After the encounter is over she seeks to retreat back to her solitude or to her Jade Dragon to further solidify the energy she acquired from the encounter.

- Men who demand a romantic relationship with the White Tigress outside the encounters, who become harsh in words or actions towards her, who encourage her to take stimulants (drugs or alcohol), who act aggressively about engaging in intercourse, or who show disinterest or laxness about her oral practices are dismissed and never seen again.

As previously mentioned, most Green Dragons are unaware that they are being seduced by a White Tigress and used for her practices. But in some cases the Green Dragon is made aware of it. For example, if the White Tigress discovers that the man has a keen interest in sexual-spiritual practices, she may choose to explain to him her reasons for having seduced him. Likewise, in cases where the man has some knowledge of these types of practices, he may become curious about her behaviors. It is then up to her discretion to explain as little or as much about it as she deems necessary.

Sometimes a Green Dragon either becomes aware that he is being watched by a Jade Dragon or is told beforehand that there will be someone watching the sexual encounter. In the case of a Green Dragon's becoming aware of the Jade Dragon's presence, the Green Dragon should remain quiet about it if he wishes to continue being with the White Tigress, for if he becomes upset or demands not to be watched she will discontinue being with him. Green Dragons that are told beforehand and agree to being watched should exercise politeness and respect, along with support of both the White Tigress and Jade Dragon.

Heavenly Vault Monastery

In regard to the manner in which traditional practices formerly occurred in China, Madame Lin recounted wonderful stories about a Taoist temple on Mount Heavenly Vault between Taihu Lake and Soochow called Heavenly Vault Monastery, where she initially experienced Illumination of the Mind. This was a very large monastery complex with more than five thousand rooms and numerous buildings and gardens spread out over hundreds of acres. The monastery functioned under the Taoist sect of Cheng-I but would host sects of other Taoist traditions as well, including White Tigresses. There were several other Taoist monasteries throughout China that welcomed the adherents of the White Tigresses—such as monasteries in the locales of Chingtao, Wanhsien, and Kuangchou—but for Madame Lin the Heavenly Vault Monastery was the most exquisite and supportive.

On several occasions, Madame Lin and her current Jade Dragon would make arrangements to stay at the monastery for one or two weeks. The abbot of the monastery would reserve a certain building far removed from the main temple grounds for the two of them to practice and live. Upon their arrival, several young men would gather, some of whom were novice monks and others who were from the village of Good Man's Bridge. Madame Lin and her Jade Dragon would interview and select nine of the men to act as her Green Dragons. Everything they needed for undisturbed and optimal practice was available to them at this monastery. There was even a private building designated for the preparation of herbs, wherein some of the oldest and most traditional formulas were prepared and stored by some of the most learned Taoist herbalists. To Madame Lin this was an absolute treasury of herbal knowledge, but, unfortunately, the Communist government later destroyed the herbal laboratory when they evicted all the monks and began using the building for military operations.

Madame Lin described their living quarters as an exquisite Sung dynasty-style building made almost entirely of lacquered wood from the nan tree, nestled neatly within a small cove on a hillside. The view from each room overlooked a grove of luxuriant pine and tall bamboo trees, all of which were accentuated by a small pond that emptied into a stream. To Madame Lin there never was any other place that could measure up to the tranquillity of the monastery, with the sounds of the wind blowing through the bamboos, the babbling of the stream, the koi fish splashing about in the pond, and the temple bells in the distance, as well as the fragrant smell of the pines and incense wafting through the air from the main temple. All parts of the environment induced a heightened sense of tranquillity and contentment.

The only disturbance Madame Lin remembered was when the

temple would conduct festivals and hundreds of pilgrims would gather to make their observances and offerings to the deities or the event being honored. On occasion one or more of these visitors wandered out along the numerous stone pathways to explore the temple grounds. When discovering the building occupied by Madame Lin and her Jade Dragon, the visitors' curiosity would get the best of them and the Jade Dragon would have to go out and politely turn them away, claiming that hermits who did not wish to be disturbed were meditating inside. This usually caused the visitors to rush away, because to disturb men of such virtue was to commit a grave sin. Madame Lin humorously noted that if some of these people knew what she was doing inside they would have never left, and a whole community of onlookers would have gathered.

The daily schedule she maintained at the monastery consisted of waking early in the morning to perform her kung fu, qigong, and Restoration Exercises. After taking a small breakfast of rice and pickled vegetables, she would take a long slow walk along the seemingly endless stone pathways among the green pines and bamboos. During these walks she donned a deep blue Tang dynasty robe, which completely concealed her figure lest she happened upon a celibate monk or pilgrim. After her walk she would sit on a small terrace with her Jade Dragon, drinking tea while conversing with him and admiring the scenery of the surrounding gardens and landscape.

At eleven o'clock in the morning two young monks would quietly approach to deliver lunch to Madame Lin and her Jade Dragon on handmade bamboo trays. The meal usually consisted of four or five dishes, mostly vegetarian with a small quantity of sliced meat. After lunch Madame Lin spent her time reading until one of her

Green Dragons, a young novice monk, arrived. At this point they retired to her bedchamber. Before engaging in any sexual practice, Madame Lin often used the afternoon appointment to receive a massage from the young monk, who was well trained in the arts of *an mo* (massage) and *tui na* (a forerunner of shiatsu).

When finished with the afternoon Green Dragon encounter Madame Lin would enter her Jade Dragon's room. He had been secretly watching them while seated on a bench behind an elaborately designed lattice screen that allowed him a close yet undetected view of the entire encounter. Retiring to his bedchamber, they would practice one or more of the Transformational Techniques or Yellow Stream methods. By late afternoon she would take a short nap or wade in the cool waters of the pond outside their dwelling.

For dinner both Madame Lin and the Jade Dragon walked to the main dining hall, an arduous and beautiful trek over various moon bridges, steep stone steps, and pathways. Before eating they would first enter the hall devoted to Hsi Wang Mu and offer incense and prayers, requesting her blessings upon their practice. Sometimes when the abbot was available, they would stay an extra hour to converse with him, as he had been a close friend of her Jade Dragon since childhood. She loved listening to them reminisce about everything but Taoism; she imagined it must have been a welcome reprieve for him to just sit and talk about mundane things, rather than about the affairs of the monastery and the training of the monks. She liked the abbot very much. He was a man in his late sixties, but he was very vibrant and young-looking, especially his eyes, which she considered clear, distinctive, and penetrating. She admired his calmness, which she thought amazing considering all

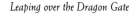

the duties he had as abbot of such a large monastery. Becoming the abbot of this wonderful monastery surely seemed a blessing to him at the time, but his vigorous devotion to keeping the monastery active and viable must have been more than wearing during those turbulent times, and little did anyone know that in just a few years the Red Tide would swarm his paradise, destroying everything. The temple was built sometime during the T'ang dynasty and restored in the Ming Dynasty by Emperor Chien Lung but later fell into disrepair. Of the five thousand compartments, only about a thousand rooms were actually maintained and a little more than a hundred and fifty monks resided there.

Upon returning to their dwelling after dinner Madame Lin and the Jade Dragon would summon another Green Dragon, and she would repeat everything with him and then with her Jade Dragon. After a late-evening bath and a short period of meditation, she would go to her bedchamber to sleep.

To Madame Lin these were the best of times, as she was young and eager to complete her Restoration Period with her first of three Jade Dragons. Her visits to Heavenly Vault Monastery were like visits to the Heavenly Immortal Abode itself, and she always felt sad when those days came to an end. She had a long family and lineage tradition connected with this monastery, as two of her aunts and several of her White Tigresses had practiced and studied there. After the destruction of the monastery, it was hard for her to accept that a place so imbued with spiritual and physical tranquillity had been destroyed, and with it Taoist monks who so openly accepted her practices—a trademark of Taoism, in which each person's view of finding the Tao is respected.

On Madame Lin's third visit to Heavenly Vault Monastery she first experienced the ultimate effects of Absorbing the Dragon's Breath and Illumination; thus she regarded the place with a special affection. Her Jade Dragon had experienced the Yellow Stream twice during their second visit—once while practicing Gazing at the Green Dragon and then again while sitting in meditation—and he stayed on, becoming a monk, after their three-year period ended.

For Madame Lin no other monastery or place of practice (*chang tao*) ever equaled the beauty and tranquillity of this monastery. After her last visit she went to live in the Shantung province, where within just a few years she was one of the many arrested by the Communist regime for sex crimes—bogus charges meant solely to embarrass the wealthy and make the Communists appear moral and concerned for public decency. Any sexual societies as well as the taking of concubines were made illegal under the new regime and were punishable by ten years in a prison work camp. Fortunately, Madame Lin escaped from having to serve her full term and went to live in Taiwan. But ever since the demise of the Heavenly Vault Monastery, she has felt that one of the most beautiful pieces of the White Tigress history had also been destroyed.

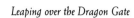

TWO

The Eight Images and Five Elements of the Jade Stem

> *All dragons reveal their power by their marks and activities;*
> *this is how a dragon can be subdued.*
> *Like winding through the crooks of a rocky grotto, the tigress knows*
> *which path leads home and those that do not.*
>
> **—White Tigress Manual**

The *White Tigress Manual* provides a correlation of various penis types with the Eight Images (*pa kua*) of the I Ching (Book of Changes), and further correlations of how each of the eight types functions within the theory of the Five Elements (*wu hsing*). Below are these definitions, so that each male reader can determine what type of penis he has and what element controls his glans penis and semen. This information can be very valuable in determining how best to revitalize, strengthen, and maintain the penis.

In order to help the reader better understand the correlations made in this section, a brief explanation is needed for how the specific trigrams indicated for each penis type are to be interpreted. A trigram is comprised of three lines, either a yin or yang line. A yang line indicates strength, and a yin line indicates weakness.

First, the Jade Stem, or penis, is comprised of three main functioning parts that determine its size: the *corpus spongiosum, corpora cavernosa*, and *glans penis*. These are explained in the section Enlarging the Glans Penis. Briefly, the corpus spongiosum is an elastic and fibrous membrane that runs from the base of the penis to the glans

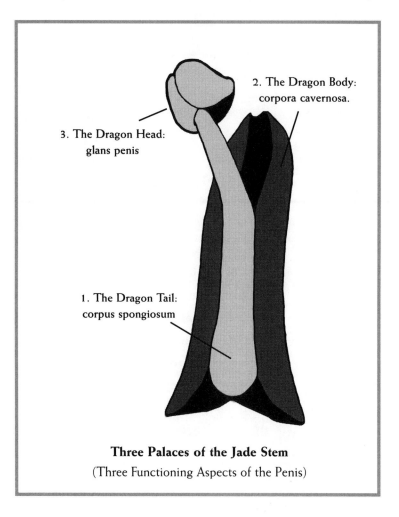

2. The Dragon Body: corpora cavernosa.

3. The Dragon Head: glans penis

1. The Dragon Tail: corpus spongiosum

Three Palaces of the Jade Stem
(Three Functioning Aspects of the Penis)

penis; the corpora cavernosa are the two side-by-side chambers that fill with blood to create the erection, and the glans penis is the head of penis. In old Chinese sex manuals these three areas of the penis are termed as shown on the diagram on page 40.

The Dragon Tail is represented by the first or bottom line of the trigram, the second or middle line represents the Dragon Body, and the third or top line represents the Dragon Head. Within each trigram image, these three lines indicate whether or not a specific penis type has a strength or weakness associated with it. Therefore, depending on which part of the penis reveals a yin aspect, strengthening that part will greatly improve not only sexual performance, but also sexual energy.

The Eight Types of Jade Stems

According to the *White Tigress Manual*, there are eight basic types of penises, each of which relates to a specific image presented in the Eight Diagrams. These are: the Heavenly Jade Stem, the Valley Jade Stem, the Fire Jade Stem, the Thunder Jade Stem, the Wind Jade Stem, the Water Jade Stem, the Mountain Jade Stem, and the Earthly Jade Stem.

Below is a brief description of each of these eight types of Jade Stems. Following this are two other correlations using the Five Elements to determine the glans penis type and semen type. All three of these correlation methods are used to better help the man revitalize, strengthen, and maintain the Jade Stem and his sexual energy.

Before moving on, note that there are four Jade Stem types that are classified as yang and four classified as yin. Yang types are invariably stronger and larger yet can cause greater health problems for the man. The yin types are invariably weaker and smaller but pose less health problems for the man. In the end, each type should be strengthened and maintained throughout a man's life so that the sexual energy remains strong, strengthening both the qi and shen.

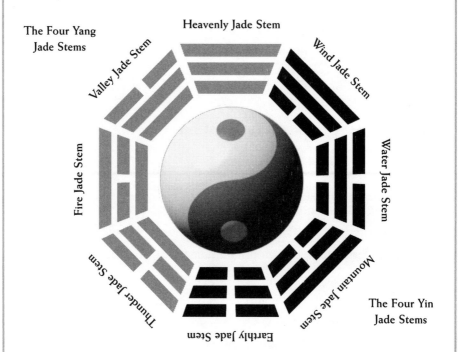

The Eight Images Representing the Eight Types of Jade Stems

The Four Yang Jade Stems

Ch'ien/Heavenly Jade Stem: T'ai Yang (Ultimate Yang)

This penis is large and broad like Heaven. It is eight inches or more in length, with a girth of at least seven inches. It is represented by three strong yang lines, meaning there is strength in all three areas of the penis. The Heavenly Jade Stem is the most attractive of all penis types, as it appears strong, smooth, and without blemishes or defects. It tends to seek long-lasting stimulation and intense orgasm.

The Heavenly Jade Stem is ruled by Horse, so the man who possesses it is likely to be attractive and have the demeanor of wanting to control females during sexual activity. He is both strong and obstinate. To attract females he primarily uses his good appearance and bold nature, as his face and head are his ruling body parts.

In terms of health, great attention must be paid to the prevention of stomach disorders; if abused or improperly maintained, this type of penis will negatively affect the qi in the stomach.

This Jade Stem will function at its best during the time of the new moon and at its worst during the full moon. The most opportune time for sexual activity is in the summer, when the sexual energy of the Heavenly Jade Stem is at its peak.

Tui/Valley Jade Stem: Shao Yang (Young Yang)

This type of penis is very wide, with a girth of seven inches or more, yet short in length (three inches or less). It is represented by two yang lines and one yin, meaning there is strength in the Dragon Tail and the Dragon Body but weakness in the Dragon Head.

The Valley Jade Stem is the most sensitive yet most penetrating of all penis types. It seeks quick stimulation, but like water running through a brook it meets many obstacles, so ejaculation is sometimes difficult.

This type of Jade Stem is ruled by the Ram, so the man who possesses it will be energetic in appearance but will have the demeanor of wandering from female to female for sexual activity; he likes to give pleasure and to rejoice. To attract females he uses words, as the mouth is his ruling body part.

In terms of health, great attention must be paid to the prevention of hand and arm disorders; if abused or improperly maintained, this type of penis will negatively affect the qi in the upper limbs.

This Jade Stem will function at its best during the time of the waxing (crescent) moon and at its worst during the waning (gibbous) moon. The most opportune time for sexual activity is in late summer, when the sexual energy of this type of penis is at its peak.

Li/Fire Jade Stem: Chung Yang (Medium Yang)

This type of penis is of medium thickness and length and tends to be bent to the left. It is seven inches or more in length and five inches in girth. It is represented by two yang lines and one yin, meaning there is strength in the Dragon Tail and the Dragon Head but weakness in the Dragon Body.

The Fire Jade Stem yearns for intense stimulation but is not long lasting. Like a burning log, that once extinguished remains hot, this Jade Stem tends to seek repeated stimulation.

This type of Jade Stem is ruled by the Phoenix, so the man who possesses it will be grand in appearance but will have the demeanor of boasting to females. He is both clinging and dependable. To attract females he sensuously stares at them, as the eyes are his ruling body part.

In terms of health, great attention must be paid to the prevention of ear disorders; if abused or improperly maintained, this type of penis will negatively affect the qi in the neck and ears.

This Jade Stem will function at its best during the time of the first half moon and at its worst during the last half moon. The most opportune time for sexual activity is in late autumn, when the sexual energy of this type of penis is at its peak.

Chen/Thunder Jade Stem: Lao Yang (Old Yang)

This type of penis is very quick to attain erection, but it does not last long. It is five inches or less in length, with a girth of five inches. It is represented by one yang line and two yin, meaning there is strength in the Dragon Tail but weaknesses in the Dragon Body and the Dragon Head.

The Thunder Jade Stem yearns only for quick stimulation and ejaculation. Like lightning in a storm, it is quick to excite but does not last.

This type of Jade Stem is ruled by the Dragon, so the man who possesses it will be charismatic in appearance and have the demeanor of promising too much to females; he is both arousing and inciting in his actions. To attract females he moves about and around them, as the feet are his ruling body part.

In terms of health, great attention must be paid to the prevention of ligament disorders; if abused or improperly maintained, this type of penis will negatively affect the qi in the muscles.

This Jade Stem will function at its best during the time of the waxing (crescent) moon and at its worst during the waning (gibbous) moon. The most opportune time for sexual activity is in late summer, when the sexual energy of this type of penis is at its peak.

The Four Yin Jade Stems

Sun/Wind Jade Stem: Lao Yin (Old Yin)
This penis type is thin, three inches or less in girth, and of medium length (six inches or less). It is represented by two yang lines and one yin, meaning there is a weakness in the Dragon Tail but strength in the Dragon Body and the Dragon Head.

The Wind Jade Stem yearns for extended and constant stimulation. Like the gusting wind, its movement is long lasting yet sporadic.

This type of Jade Stem is ruled by the Rooster, so the man who possesses it will be honest and fair in appearance and have the demeanor of being too gentle with females; he is both penetrating and scattered in his actions. To attract females he draws close to them, as the thighs are his ruling body part.

In terms of health, great attention must be paid to the prevention of tendon disorders; if abused or improperly maintained, this type of penis will negatively affect the qi in the bones and joints.

This Jade Stem will function at its best during the time of the waning (crescent) moon and at its worst during the waxing (gibbous) moon. The most opportune time for sexual activity is in early spring, when the sexual energy of this type of penis is at its peak.

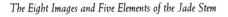

K'an/Water Jade Stem: Chung Yin (Medium Yin)
This type of penis is of medium thickness and length and tends to be bent to the right. It is six inches or more in length, with a girth of four inches or less. It is represented by two yang lines and one yin, meaning there is strength in the Dragon Body but weakness in the Dragon Tail and the Dragon Head. The Water Jade Stem is the most difficult to stimulate, as it is slow to attain erection and ejaculation. Therefore, it yearns for slowness and patience in stimulation.

This type of Jade Stem is ruled by the Boar, so the man who possesses it will be dangerous in appearance and have the demeanor of being too mysterious with females; he is both perilous and deep in his actions. To attract females he intently listens to them, as the ears are his ruling body part.

In terms of health, great attention must be paid to the prevention of eye disorders; if abused or improperly maintained, this type of penis will negatively affect the qi in the eyes and central nervous system.

This Jade Stem will function at its best during the time of the waning half moon and at its worst during the waxing half moon. The most opportune time for sexual activity is in spring, when the sexual energy of this type of penis is at its peak.

Ken/Mountain Jade Stem: Shao Yin (Young Yin)
This type of penis is very long, eight inches or more, and of medium thickness (5 inches). It is represented by two yin lines and one yang, meaning there is strength in the Dragon Head but weakness in the Dragon Body and the Dragon Tail.

The Mountain Jade Stem yearns for frequent erection and attention. It is long lasting but slow to ejaculate, so it requires intense and prolonged stimulation.

This type of Jade Stem is ruled by the Dog, so the man who possesses it will be loyal and calm in appearance and have the demeanor of being too at ease with females. He is capturing and supportive in his actions. To attract females he takes care of things for them, as the hands are his ruling body part.

In terms of health, great attention must be paid to the prevention of oral disorders; if abused or improperly maintained, this type of penis will negatively affect the qi in the neck and face.

This Jade Stem will function at its best during the time of the waning (gibbous) moon and at its worst during the waxing (crescent) moon. The most opportune time for sexual activity is in early winter, when the sexual energy of this type of penis is at its peak.

K'un/Earthly Jade Stem: T'ai Yin (Ultimate Yin)

This type of penis is thin in both length and girth. It is four inches or less in length and three inches or less in girth. It is represented by three yin lines, meaning there is weakness in the Dragon Tail, the Dragon Body, and the Dragon Head.

The Earthly Jade Stem does not actively seek stimulation or ejaculation but responds when stimulation occurs. It tends to seek prolonged stimulation with mild intensity.

This type of Jade Stem is ruled by the Ox, so the man who possesses it will be yielding and harmless in appearance and have the demeanor of being too devoted and stubborn with females. He is both receptive and giving in his actions. To attract females he nourishes and cares for them, as the stomach is his ruling body part.

In terms of health, great attention must be paid to the prevention of head disorders; if abused or improperly maintained, this type of penis will negatively affect the qi in the brain and central nervous system.

This Jade Stem will function at its best during the time of the full moon and at its worst during the new moon. The most opportune time for sexual activity is in winter, when the sexual energy of this type of penis is at its peak.

The Five Element Correspondences of the Glans Penis

The Horse Head (Metal)

Ruled by the Horse, this type of glans penis is broad and muscular in appearance with a very prominent rim at the base of the glans. Its secretions resemble the texture and feel of saliva, which benefits a female's immune system when ingested.

The Boar Head (Water)

Ruled by the Boar, this type of glans penis is broad and flat in appearance with very little accentuation of the rim at the base of the penis. Its secretions resemble the texture and feel of semen, which benefits the female's endocrine system when ingested.

The Five Element Correspondences of the Glans Penis

Ram Head
(Fire Element)

Rooster Head
(Wood Element)

Ox Head
(Earth Element)

Boar Head
(Water Element)

Horse Head
(Metal Element)

The Rooster Head (Wood)

Ruled by the Rooster, this type of glans penis is thin and elongated in appearance with a smooth tapering of the rim at the base of the glans. Its secretions resemble the texture and feel of perspiration, which benefits the female's circulatory system when ingested.

The Ram Head (Fire)

Ruled by the Ram, this type of glans penis is pointed and slim in appearance with a curved rim at the base of the glans. Its secretions resemble the texture and feel of mucus, which benefits the female's digestive system when ingested.

The Ox Head (Earth)

Ruled by the Ox, this type of glans penis is very broad and thick in appearance with a thick accentuation of the rim at the base of the glans. Its secretions resemble the texture and feel of tears, which benefits the female's central nervous system when ingested.

The Five Element Correspondences of the Semen

Below are listed the five types of semen (ching), two of which are considered the ideal or positive types (White Tiger and Yellow Horse) and the remaining three considered not ideal or negative types (Black Tortoise, Green Dragon, and Red Phoenix).

Each man is born with a certain type of semen (inherited from his parents), so some males naturally have ideal or healthy semen and some do not. The Taoist refers to this as the "Before Heaven" conditions, which apply to all the physical and mental characteristics we are born with. A male may damage his inherent semen type through a variety of self-abuses: excessive dissipation, poor diet, alcohol or drugs, poor exercise, mental fanaticism, and so on. The Taoists refer to this as the "After Heaven" conditions. Thus each male is born with a certain positive or negative condition of his semen (Before Heaven), and each male is capable of either maintaining a positive condition or changing a negative one through various restoration methods: exercises, herbs, and disciplines.

All males periodically undergo changes in both their semen quality and quantity. Sometimes semen can even appear as a combination of different types. The type of semen a man has depends entirely how he treats himself both physically and mentally. The methods of the Jade Dragon are meant to aid in the maintenance, to the best degree possible, of both the quality and quantity of White Tiger or Yellow Horse semen.

The purpose of this section is to allow the reader to determine what type of semen he has and to identify which of the five elements (Metal, Water, Wood, Fire, and Earth) is associated with it. The significance of these five elements it is not the actual element itself, but rather the "activity" of the element. For example, Metal is strong and penetrating, Water is soft and moving, Wood is pliable and spreading, Fire is hot and dispersing, and Earth is stable and nourishing.

Each man can change his semen type from a negative one to a positive one or be able to maintain the positive semen type he was

Red Phoenix Ching
(Fire Element)
Fire is created by Wood
Fire destroys Metal
Fire complements Earth

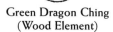

Green Dragon Ching
(Wood Element)
Wood is created by Water
Wood destroys Earth
Wood complements Fire

Yellow Horse Ching
(Earth Element)
Earth is created by Fire
Earth destroys Water
Earth complements Metal

Black Tortoise Ching
(Water Element)
Water is created by Metal
Water destroys Fire
Water complements Wood

White Tiger Ching
(Metal Element)
Metal is created by Earth
Metal destroys Wood
Metal complements Water

The Five Element Correspondences of the Semen

born with. The restorations or stablizations of semen (described in detail in chapter 4) primarily lies in disciplines of taking the proper herbs, exercising the penis and testicles, moderation in ejaculation, proper diet, and learning to have a healthy and stress-free lifestyle. Through these disciplines a man can acquire or maintain the positive semen conditions of either the White Tiger or Yellow Horse types.

White Tiger Ching (Metal)

The element of Metal is the strongest, like the element of Earth (enduring and solid). White Tiger Ching is created by the element of Earth (revealed by its thick consistency) and complements Water (nourishing the liquidity of semen). Metal destroys the element of Wood, which has the negative characteristic of burning or rotting, so this semen remains strong. For these reasons the White Tiger Ching (semen) is considered a positive semen type.

Symptoms: Hard, spurting ejaculations, pure white, thick consistency, cool in temperature, slightly pungent taste, mildly spoiled odor.

Cause: This type of semen is the result of heredity as well as maintaining moderate ejaculation frequency, good diet, good spirits, and frequent exercise. Healthy semen of this type is nourishing to the kidneys, genitals, and bones. Since Earth is the element that creates Metal, the most effective remedies for maintaining and strengthening this type of semen is through eating sweet organic foods (such as fruits), drinking fragrant teas and juices, and eating cooked millet, as well as practicing the Jade Dragon methods for restoration (herbs and exercises).

Defects: If semen of this type is depleted or damaged, it can negatively affect the liver, eyes, and ligaments. Since Fire is the element that destroys Metal, the most harmful foods for this semen type are bitter and fried foods. Since Wood is the element that contends with Metal, the emotion of anger should be avoided.

Black Tortoise Ching (Water)

Black Tortoise Ching is created by Metal but is weakened by itself, as Water causes Metal to rust and deteriorate, so it will cause the semen to be weakened. Water complements the element of Wood, but also causes Wood to rot and decay, making the semen putrid. Water also destroys Fire, taking the heat and consistency from the semen. For these reasons the Black Tortoise Ching (semen) is considered a negative semen type.

Symptoms: Dribbling ejaculations, clear color, thin consistency, cool temperature, slightly salty taste, mildly putrid odor.

Cause: Frequent ejaculation, bad diet or excessive alcohol consumption, and poor exercise.

Defects: If depleted or damaged, semen of this type can negatively affect the heart, ears, and arteries. But if kept healthy or strengthened, it is nourishing to the liver, eyes, and ligaments. Since Metal creates Water it is best to follow the restoration methods given under White Tiger (above) to change into White Tiger (Metal) semen.

Green Dragon Ching (Wood)

The element of Wood is not enduring. Green Dragon Ching is created by Water but is weakened by itself, as Wood rots and deteriorates, so it will cause the semen to be weakened. Wood complements the element of Fire, but Fire burns Wood, making the semen inconsistent in both temperature and consistency. Wood also destroys

Earth, taking the thickness and endurance from the semen. For these reasons the Green Dragon Ching (semen) is considered a negative semen type.

Symptoms: Streaming ejaculations, hint of gray color, stringy consistency, moderate temperature, slightly sour taste, and mildly rancid odor.

Cause: Fluctuating frequency of ejaculation, mental stress and uneasiness, and infrequent or poor exercise.

Defects: If depleted or damaged, semen of this type can negatively affect the kidneys, genitals, and bones. When kept healthy or strengthened, it is nourishing to the heart, ears, and arteries. Since Water creates Wood it is best to follow the restoration methods given under White Tiger (above) to change it into White Tiger (Metal) semen, and because Wood destroys Earth it will not be useful to attempt to change it into Yellow Horse (Earth) semen.

Red Phoenix Ching (Fire)

The element of Fire is not enduring. Red Phoenix Ching is created by Wood and therefore is weakened by itself, as Fire burns Wood, so it will cause the semen to dry up. Fire complements the element of Earth, which gives it some strength, especially temperature wise. Fire also destroys Metal, taking away the thick consistency from the semen. For these reasons the Red Phoenix Ching (semen) is considered a negative semen type.

Symptoms: Spraying, hint of pink color, lumpy consistency, very hot temperature, slightly bitter taste, mildly scorched odor.

Cause: Excessive ejaculations, excessive fantasizing, sporadic exercise.

Defects: If depleted or damaged, semen of this type can negatively affect the lungs, mouth, and skin. But if kept healthy or strengthened, it is nourishing to the spleen, nose, and muscles. Since Wood creates Fire it is best to follow the restoration methods given under Yellow Horse (below) to change into Yellow Horse (Earth) semen, because Fire complements Earth.

Yellow Horse Ching (Earth)

The element of Earth is the most enduring, like the element of Metal. Yellow Horse Ching is created by the element of Fire (passion and heat) and complements Metal (giving it even greater strength). Earth absorbs the element of Water, which it uses to nourish itself. For these reasons the Yellow Horse Ching (semen) is considered a positive semen type.

Symptoms: Slow oozing, hint of yellow color, globby consistency, neutral temperature, slightly sweet taste, mildly fragrant odor.

Cause: This type of semen is the result of heredity as well as maintaining moderate ejaculation frequency, good diet, good spirits, and frequent exercise. Healthy semen of this type is nourishing to the spleen, genitals, and muscles. Since Fire is the element that creates Earth, the most effective remedies for maintaining or creating this type of semen is through eating organic vegetables, drinking green teas and wine, and eating cooked rice, as well as practicing the Jade Dragon methods for restoration (herbs and exercises).

Defects: If semen of this type is depleted or damaged, it can negatively affect the kidneys, genitals, and bones. But if it is kept healthy or strengthened, it is nourishing to the lungs, mouth, and skin.

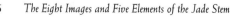

THREE

Revitalization
of the Dragon Ching

龍
精

> *The elixir of immortality, you need not beg for it from others.*
> *The eight images are within your palms,*
> *The five elements are residing within you.*
> *Understanding this, the spirits will guide you to immortality.*
>
> **—White Tigress Manual**

The first and most important task of any self-cultivator, regardless of his chosen tradition or practice, is to either maintain or revitalize his health. Good health is rooted in a person's sexual energy and capabilities. This does not mean that a person must be sexual to be in good health, but that each person is designed biologically to be sexual and the very fabric of our physical well-being is based on our ability to be sexually active. For example, when we are suffering from an illness or disease we normally lose our sex drive; when we recover from the illness and regain our health we experience sexual desire. The Taoists understood clearly that without optimum sexual energy (ching) there is insufficient internal energy to forge what they call the Elixir of Immortality, which is a result of optimum accumulation and refinement of the Three Treasures.

To make an analogy, the ching is like the fuse on a stick of dynamite, the qi is like the explosive material, and the shen is like the actual force of exploding dynamite. Without the fuse to ignite the dynamite the explosive material can not function. It is the same in the human body; without sufficient ching the body can not produce sufficient qi, and without sufficient qi the shen cannot be activated. This is the reason we find in so many spiritual traditions for revitalizing the adherents' internal and external energy. In activities from yoga to martial arts, there is always great emphasis on acquiring and maintaining optimum health. For the Jade Dragon, then, it is paramount to maintain sexual energy, a well-functioning Jade Stem, and beneficial semen. Hence, the Jade Dragon undertakes the practice of specialized Jade Stem exercises and the ingestion of various herbs to ensure the development of his sexual energy and performance.

The first concern of any male wanting to engage in these practices is strong ching (sexual energy), which is based on him having a fully functioning Jade Stem and beneficial semen for the White Tigress. Without these, the practice is hampered and less beneficial to both parties.

In some Taoist practices, ching is accumulated by males simply by retaining semen and discarding sexual activity altogether, in other words, by becoming celibate. The effectiveness of celibacy is not denied here, but keep in mind that celibacy within a monk's or nun's spiritual cultivation is done for different reasons. Celibacy is usually undertaken to purify the mind, and so the focus is on developing the spirit to be strong enough to stimulate the ching and qi. The Jade Dragon's practices develop the ching so that it will be strong enough to stimulate the qi and shen. It is simply a matter of looking at different sides of the same coin. Celibacy can in some instances be dangerous and injurious to a male's health, just as overindulgence in sex can be destructive. Biologically, however, all males are born with the function of semen ejaculation, and they will need to ejaculate periodically to maintain physical and mental well-being.

There is some truth to the idea that it is not the size of the penis that matters but how it is used during sex that makes all the difference to a woman. However, it is also true that a thicker penis often gives more satisfaction to a woman. Larger girth (circumference) is preferable even during oral sex, mainly because it visually expresses to her the male's virility. Length is not important in this regard, as a man with a thicker penis, especially an enlarged glans penis, sexually excites a woman more than a man with a long penis. In terms of fellatio, an enlarged glans penis provides several benefits. It affords more surface area in which the woman can stimulate the man with her tongue and mouth, and it stimulates the inside of her mouth in order to more abundantly produce saliva, a very necessary part of the White Tigress's practice. A thicker penis is also able to create more sensation in the vagina and on the clitoris during intercourse. Likewise, a man with a thicker penis will also experience more sensation when inside the woman's vagina.

Men should keep in mind that women are capable of passing an eight-pound or larger baby through their vaginas, so the average penis really isn't all that intimidating to them. On average, most men are 5.5 inches when erect, with a girth of about 4 inches. A large penis falls into the category of 7 inches or more, with a girth of 6 inches or more. Remember that it is the girth of a penis that is more useful during sex. If a man's penis is too long most women do not enjoy intercourse when he thrusts deeply into them. But when a woman is fully stimulated, a wider penis can feel far better to her than a thinner one.

According to the comments White Tigresses have made to me, females prefer males with a strong, bigger, and especially thicker penis. Most men would like to have penises that are a little longer and thicker. It is often said that size does not matter, but in honesty I think the consensus for both females and males is that, on a purely sexual level, size does matter. When love is factored into the situation, the issue of size becomes much less important.

Men gain more self-confidence when they can perform sexually to their fullest potential. They like to have more erections, to maintain the erections longer, and to ejaculate more semen during climax. This is not just a macho male desire, it is an inherent psychological need within most males to feel sexually powerful—just as most women desire to be thought of as beautiful and alluring. Generally, a man loves to hear from his partner that she loves his penis, and that he performs well sexually.

No man should ever just sit back and think he is sexually perfect, because there is always room for improvement and the older he gets the more help he needs to maintain his sexual prowess. It is only common sense that men would want to accomplish all this naturally and safely, and that is exactly what the Jade Dragon methods are: natural and safe.

Medical science thought for years that penis size was purely

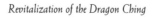

hereditary and nothing could be done to increase it. Most ancient cultures, however, such as those in China, the Middle East, and South America, created methods and discovered herbs for increasing the size of the penis and enhancing sexual performance. These methods and herbs have worked within these cultures for hundreds and, in some cases, thousands of years. The truth is that your penis can be enlarged, and your sexual prowess can be increased.

The penis is primarily a mass of erectile tissue comprised of three fibrous cylindrical tubes placed side by side, forming the shaft of the penis. When these fill with blood an erection is produced.

The two largest chambers on the right and left sides of the penis shaft are called the corpora cavernosa, and the smaller one, in the center of the penis shaft, is called corpus spongiosum. The length and girth of the penis are primarily determined by the corpora cavernosa, the two chambers that intake blood for producing an erection. Through herbs and exercises that stretch and expand these two chambers of the penis, the length and girth can be enlarged.

Also determining the length of the penis is the corpus spongiosum, which is very elastic and fibrous and runs through the center of the penis shaft from the base (beneath the pubic bone, called the bulb of the corpus spongiosum) to the glans penis (the head). Again, the effects of the herbs and the special exercises stretch the corpus spongiosum so that the length of the penis is increased.

These chambers are fed blood by three main paths, two of which, the central arteries, run directly through the corpora cavernosa. These arteries provide the blood needed to fill the chambers. The third path, the dorsal vein, runs over the top of the penis and feeds numerous veins and capillaries throughout the penis shaft.

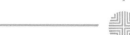

The herbs encourage increased blood flow through all these blood vessels, making it possible to expand the penis with exercise, very much like the process of expanding and strengthening any body muscle.

Once the herbs have been ingested and have taken effect (about thirty minutes), it is time to exercise the penis with the Nine Jade Dragon Exercises. This specific program of exercises stretches, expands, and strengthens the penis chambers to allow more blood into the penis, thus making it bigger. These exercises are the very crux of the Jade Dragon methods.

The three more modern medically proven male genital stimulant herbs of saw palmetto, yohimbe, and ginseng can enhance blood flow to the penis, expand the blood vessels in the penis, enlarge the corpora cavernosa in the penis shaft, and increase sexual energy. However, Taoists centuries ago developed herbal formulas which, in my opinion, were much more effective than just the ingestion of a single herbal substance, as will be shown later under the heading Ancient Herbal Formulas for Sexual Revitalization (see page 64). When taken correctly, these herbs, in conjunction with proper exercises, can have profound effects on the size and performance of the penis.

Normally, a man gets an erection, climaxes, and the sexual encounter is over. Nothing he does during the sexual act helps him increase the size of his penis. The chambers and vessels of the penis are not exercised to increase mass through normal sexual or masturbatory activities. Normal sexual activity can be seen as analogous to a person who is very active every day but doesn't develop a body builder's physique. A body builder develops muscle groups individually through intense focused weight lifting. The Nine Jade Dragon Exercises teach you to strengthen and enlarge the penis muscle.

The Jade Dragon methods utilize herbal stimulation to increase blood flow, expand the blood vessels, and enlarge the corpora cavernosa. Then specific exercises are performed so that the penis can gradually accept more blood. Every day the penis is expanded to accommodate more blood. Since erections are simply the engorgement of the penis chambers with blood, the more room you make for the blood, the larger, longer, and thicker the penis becomes. There is nothing complicated about these methods; all it takes is the right herbs, the right exercises, and a little discipline.

It is not enough to just have a bigger penis; you should also have the energy and staying power to use it. Nothing is worse than not to achieve a complete erection during sex or to lack the ability to maintain it until climax. It is also important to be able to climax at least two or three times during a sexual encounter. Granted, sometimes once is enough, but other times it is good to be multiorgasmic. After thirty years of age, achieving multiple orgasms becomes increasingly difficult.

Many men are too quick to climax and leave their partner feeling unfulfilled and frustrated. Acquiring long-lasting erections and consecutive erections during a sexual encounter is very important for men. Sexual research has shown that a man climaxes normally within four minutes of stimulation to his penis, and a woman normally climaxes within twelve minutes. So for a man really to be a good lover, he needs not only to maintain his erection longer, but also to be multiorgasmic.

The more semen a man ejaculates while climaxing, the longer

his orgasm. Therefore, increasing the quantity of semen is very important. To the woman, a man who ejaculates a large amount of semen is seen as being very virile. During intercourse some women love the feel of their partner ejecting semen into them; it provides a wonderful sensation. Also, during oral sex many Tigresses, and I assume many women in general as well, complain if the man only ejaculates a small amount after all her efforts to bring him to climax; she may feel cheated or may think she did not satisfy him properly.

Another male sexual problem is bad-tasting or watery semen. Obviously, a partner would not like bad-tasting semen, and clear, watery semen does not project the same image of virility as thick, white semen does. In medical terms, clear, watery semen is a sign of either illness, alcoholism, or excessive dissipation. In any case, the Nine Jade Dragon Exercises will greatly benefit both the odor of the semen and the consistency, making it thicker, better smelling, and greater in quantity.

Ancient Herbal Formulas for Sexual Revitalization

In the *White Tigress Manual* various herbal formulas are given so the Jade Dragon can easily achieve three goals: increase the size of his Jade Stem, acquire more sexual prowess, and improve the quality and quantity of his ejaculation. The herbal formula given for enlarging the penis and increasing sexual stamina is called Joyful Dragon and is used in combination with an ointment called Dragon King and the calisthenics called the Nine Jade Dragon Exercises. The combination of these three methods would ensure he fully achieved all three goals.

The actual process of mixing these formulas should only be performed by a competent herbalist, as they are quite powerful and very effective. The following are several useful Chinese herbal formulas.

JOYFUL DRAGON FORMULA

3 grams Yuan chih *(Polygala japonica)*

3 grams T'u szu tzu *(Cuscuta japonica)*

4 grams She ch'uang tzu *(Cridium japonica)*

3 grams Wu wei tzu *(Schizandra sinesis)*

3 grams Jen shen *(Panax ginseng)*

3 grams Jou tsung jung *(Boschniakia glabra)*

Take the formula in pill or tea form three times a day for nine consecutive days, then take as needed.

The formula stimulates blood flow to the penis, thus expanding the corpora cavernosa, stimulating the growth of the bulb of the corpus spongiosum (which causes it to lengthen), causing the increased production of semen and the frequency and prolongation of erections, while also encouraging multiple ejaculations.

DRAGON KING OINTMENT

3 grams Jou tsung jung *(Boschniakia glabra)*

2 grams Hai tsao (Sea Grass)

9 fluid ounces Lu kan cha (Deer Liver Extract)

Apply the ointment to the outer surface of the Jade Stem three times a day for forty-five days or until the the Jade Stem's size has reached its maximum (usually two to three inches of added length and one to two inches of added girth).

The herbs in this ointment cause the skin of the penis to attract increased blood flow in the dorsal veins, arteries, and capillaries, thus causing the two corpora cavernosa chambers and the glans penis to swell. The ointment is normally used once when performing the Nine Jade Dragon Exercises, and then twice without accompanying exercises. After the ointment has been applied three times, completely wash the ointment off the penis with clean, warm water.

DRAGON HORN FORMULA

4 grams Hsien ts'ao (Immortal Grass)

4 grams Yuan chih (*Polygala japonica*)

4 grams Wu wei tzu (*Schizandra sinesis*)

4 grams Po tzu jen (*Cedar Seeds*)

4 grams Jou tsung jung (*Boschniakia glabra*)

4 grams Ch'e ch'ien tzu (*Plantago major*)

4 grams T'u szu tzu (*Cuscuta japonica*)

4 grams Jen shen (*Panax ginseng*)

This formula has many benefits, especially for men in their late forties and older. The Jade Stem will enlarge one inch in both length and girth, and erections will come much more easily when one is engaged sexually with a woman. The formula prevents the erection from shrinking during sex and greatly increases semen production, and it also cures nocturnal emissions, excess urination, and aches in the middle of the back.

Although the formula does not need to be taken every day, one should do so initially for a month or two, until the effects are readily apparent. The formula is either fashioned into small pills or taken as a tea. Thereafter, the formula can be ingested as needed for a week or two, until the effects return again. However, since the

Dragon Horn Formula and the Joyful Dragon Formula contain some of the same herbs, the two should not be taken simultaneously. Most Jade Dragons take the Joyful Dragon Formula until the maximum results are achieved and then use the Dragon Horn Formula.

Modern-Day Herbs That Revitalize Sexual Energy

In addition to the herbal formulas listed above, a man might wish to take the more readily available and popular herbs used for stimulating sexual energy and alleviating problems of the prostate: ginseng, yohimbe, and saw palmetto. Keep in mind that these herbs will be far more effective if taken in extract form. Below is a brief explanation of each of the herbs.

Ginseng

Ginseng, or *ren shen* in Chinese, is called the "king of herbs." Ginseng is revered for its ability to impart clarity and awareness to its users. In the first recorded Chinese treatise on herbs, the legendary emperor Shen Nung said: "Ginseng is a tonic to the five viscera, quieting the animal spirits, stabilizing the soul, preventing fear, expelling the vicious energies, brightening the eye and improving vision, opening up the heart, benefiting the understanding, and if taken for some time will invigorate the body and prolong life."

Ginseng root is said to aid in dispersing qi to the meridians and organs. Its name means "essence of the earth in the form of a man." The chief constituents of ginseng are long-chain polysaccharides, saponins, ginsenins, panoxic acid, panaxin, panaquilon, minerals, and some B vitamins. More than twenty-eight of the ginsenosides (a type of saponin) discovered in research the past few years have been used in studies that prove ginseng's great value to health and long life.

There are three major kinds of ginseng: Chinese (including the Siberian variety), American, and Korean. Of the Chinese herb, there are three general types: yi sun, shiu chu, and kirin. The roots of yi sun, which are very rare and quite expensive in the United States, are dug up when very young in the wild and are transplanted to cultivated beds until they reach maturity. They are then sold. These are the most potent roots available, except for wild mature roots, which are essentially unattainable.

The shiu chu roots are usually five or six years old and are probably the best deal, costing under ten dollars an ounce. Kirin is the lowest quality ginseng and is usually used for extractions or capsules. There are also many roots from specific Chinese districts that have become well known, such as ji lin.

The roots of American and Asian ginseng are considered quite distinct in their actions. White American ginseng, being more yin, reduces the heat of the lungs and respiratory systems and is considered best for improving sexual dysfunctions.

Saponins are considered to be the chief constituents of ginseng, but many other substances in the roots are also important. The ability of saponins to aid in reducing stress and their action as adaptogens has brought ginseng into the spotlight of modern herb consumers and has spurred much research. In my reading of various translated Russian and Chinese research on ginseng, it has been suggested that these saponins, or ginsenosides, are analgesic, anti-inflammatory, tranquilizing, hypotensive, a regulator of blood sugar, an aid to the digestion, and also antipsychotic and anticonvulsant.

In addition, ginseng has a beneficial effect on the heart and circulatory system, modulating not only blood pressure but also cholesterol. It stimulates the secretion of pepsin and relieves indigestion and gas. Ginseng is generally used for its tonic and adaptogenic benefits and its ability to increase strength and energy; it has also been used to encourage longevity. Taoists in China have used it for hundreds of years for quieting the spirit. The Chinese consider ginseng the "miracle herb," as it is especially good for treating ailments of the reproductive organs (including the prostate) and kidneys. In Russia, ginseng is recommended to people over the age of forty in an annual six-week program.

Much research remains to be done on ginseng but men who take it claim a higher level of physical energy and greater sexual potency. Typically, one is advised to take American white ginseng for increasing sexual energy and Chinese red ginseng for increasing semen quantity.

The reader must use some precautions when taking any herbal remedies. Just because herbal remedies are natural or organic does not mean they cannot produce negative side effects. Westerners, unfortunately, often have the idea that "more is better," and that is certainly not the case with prescription drugs or with herbal remedies. As a general rule, herbal remedies should not be taken for more than forty-five days on a daily basis. After that, one should stop taking the herb for at least two weeks before ingesting daily again, and then the remedy should be used only if needed.

Yohimbe

Yohimbe originates from the inner bark of the tree *Pausinystalia yohimbe*. This herb is considered the only credible natural sensual stimulant and sexual enhancer by the *Physician's Desk Reference*. The only substances approved by the FDA for the treatment of impotence are yohimbe and Viagra. Of the two, yohimbe is preferable because it is herbal, ten times cheaper, needs no medical prescription, and does not have the heart risk that Viagra carries.

Yohimbe has three actions that make it useful and powerful as a sexual stimulant: (1) it expands the blood vessels in the extremities of the body—the head, hands, feet, and genitals—which increases blood flow to the corpus cavernosa; (2) it inhibits and reduces the effects of hormones that constrict blood vessels, hormones that typically increase as we grow older; and (3) it increases the production of norepinephrine and adrenaline, both of which are essential to both erections and sexual stimulation.

Saw Palmetto

Saw palmetto is the fifth most popular herb on the market. The berries of the plant have been used by Native Americans for centuries as a general tonic and a cure for impotence. Research in Europe during the 1980s showed that saw palmetto was very effective in curing benign prostatic hyperplasia (BPH), a noncancerous growth of the prostate gland.

Experts estimate that about half of all men over fifty suffer from some form of prostate dysfunction, and around ten million men suffer from BPH. In a study of more than one thousand males suffering from BPH, saw palmetto cured two-thirds of the test group, which was an even higher result than that of prostatic surgery.

Saw palmetto is used to not only keep the urethra from becoming pinched during aging, but also to ensure adequate blood flow to both the prostate and the penis. It is important to keep the urethra open to accomodate the increased amount of semen that will be produced as these herbs and exercises increase sexual prowess.

The Nine Jade Dragon Exercises

It is not absolutely necessary to take any of the previously described herbs or formulas in order to perform the exercises presented below, but using both herbs and exercises is advisable for maximum effect.

Preliminary Treatments

After taking the herbs, wait approximately thirty minutes and then begin the following regimen:

- Remove all clothing from the lower body so that nothing constricts your movements.
- Soak the entire penis shaft (but not the groin) in warm water for three minutes. The water should be warmer than lukewarm but not so hot that you can't touch it, close to the temperature of warm shower water. This will help draw more blood into the penis and relax it as well.
- All the exercises should be done sitting upright on the edge of a chair.

- For all the self-massage techniques use an oil (or the Dragon King Ointment) to help make the actions easier and smoother.

Dragon Pressing Its Body

This is an acupressure exercise for strengthening erections. The exercise will ensure that sufficient blood flow and qi will reach the genital area for the following exercises.

Rub the area three inches below your navel with your right palm clockwise thirty-six times, and then clockwise with your right thumb thirty-six times on the same area.

Press hard with your thumbs three inches above the medial of the ankle, slightly behind the tibia. Press hard in and out thirty-six times on both legs.

Press hard with your thumbs three inches below the kneecap and one inch to the lateral side of the tibia. Press hard in and out thirty-six times.

With your palms massage vigorously upward along the legs to the groin area.

Dragon Wagging Its Tail

This method consists of slapping the penis head against each of the thighs. This draws increased blood into the head of the penis and desensitizes the penis so it won't ejaculate during the remainder of the exercises.

Place the right hand below the groin and press in slightly on the perineum (the space between the anus and penis) with the middle and index fingers. Hold the other fingers up and away from the area.

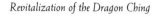

Position the left hand so that the thumb and index fingers completely encircle the base of the penis and the rest of the fingers lie along the shaft pointing toward the penis head. Slap the head of the penis against the left thigh thirty-six times. Then reverse the position of the hands and slap the penis on the right thigh thirty-six times. The slapping should be moderate and slow. Do not slap so hard that the penis feels a sting, but do not slap so soft that a sound isn't produced.

Dragon Twisting a Pillar

This method consists of twisting and pulling on the penis shaft. The benefit is that the penis begins stretching and loosening all three of the blood chambers.

Hold the base of the penis firmly with the index finger and thumb of the right hand, with the remaining fingers resting on the testicles. Bring the left hand over the penis and grasp the shaft firmly with the index finger and thumb, as in the slapping method above. Twist and pull your left hand up to the underside of the glans penis thirty-six times. Then reverse the position of your hands and twist and pull with the right hand thirty-six times.

Dragon Pressing Its Head

This method consists of squeezing and pulling the penis. This exercise aids in bringing more blood into the three chambers and glans penis. It also helps in increasing the penis's girth.

Hold the base of the penis firmly with the right hand, as in the previous exercise. Press the thumb and index finger of the left hand firmly against the front and back of the penis. As if squeezing toothpaste from a tube, bring the hand up just below the head of the penis and hold it there firmly. Use some force to try to flex and expand the muscle of the glans penis; do this nine times. Repeat the series thirty-six times, holding the penis firmly with the left hand, and then switch hands and flex thirty-six times, this time while holding the penis with the right hand.

Dragon Stretching Its Claws

This exercise is an extension of the previous one and is primarily performed to fully stretch the three chambers. In this technique, you pull down and back with one hand, while pulling out and up with the other, as if pulling the penis apart.

Hold the base of the penis with the right hand, as in the previous exercises. Then take the left hand and grasp somewhat firmly along the underside of the glans penis with the index and thumb.

Simultaneously pull outward and up with the left hand and down and back with the right hand, as if pulling the penis apart. Do this thirty-six times, then switch the position of the hands and perform another thirty-six repetitions.

Dragon Holding Its Breath

This exercise is primarily used for lengthening the penis and enlarging the glans penis. It entails both squeezing and holding blood into the head of the penis.

Hold the base of the penis firmly with the right index finger and thumb. Using the left index finger and thumb, grip the underside of the glans penis, pulling the penis slightly outward and up. Next, squeeze the penis shaft, drawing blood into the glans penis so that it enlarges slightly. Hold this position and your breath for a count of nine, and then release the pressure of the left hand. Do this three times, then change the position of the hands and do another three repetitions.

Dragon Entering the Cave
This technique is primarily used for expanding the width of the penis. It makes use of the squeezing and flattening of the penis shaft from the base up to the glans penis.

Place both thumbs and index fingers at the base of the penis shaft, with the thumbs on top of the shaft and the index fingers below. With firm back and forth motions, squeeze and flatten the penis all the way up the shaft to the underside of the glans penis. Repeat this thirty-six times.

Dragon Entering the Bamboo Stalk
This is a method for widening the penis shaft. It makes use of rolling the penis shaft between the two palms of the hands.

Place the palms of both hands along each side of the penis shaft. Starting from the base of the penis, vigorously roll and exert inward pressure on the penis, moving the hands upward along the shaft to the underside of the glans penis. Once at the top, bring the hands down to the base and begin rolling again. Repeat this thirty-six times.

Dragon Stroking Its Whiskers
This is a method for enlarging the glans penis and for lengthening the penis shaft. It makes use of a rolling of the palm over the glans penis.

Hold the base of the penis firmly with the right index finger and thumb. Swipe the left palm firmly over the glans penis, moving from the top to the back of the penis shaft. While swiping, pull, press, and stretch down as far as possible without causing pain. Pull, press, and stretch the penis to the right side thirty-six times.

Switch the hands so that the left hand is holding the base of the penis and repeat the pulling, pressing, and stretching of the penis to the left side thirty-six times.

Concluding Treatments

The following treatments should be done in conjunction with the Nine Jade Dragon Exercises; the treatments are usually performed after the exercises.

Dragon Pearl Testicle Massage

Massaging the testicles will help the production of testosterone, strengthen erections, increase the seminal fluids, and heighten your sexual energy. It is essential that you do not disregard these exercises, as they are crucial to the benefits of and development prompted by the Nine Jade Dragon Exercises. Do these massages immediately after the exercises.

Massaging the Seminal Ducts

Hold the testicles, using the thumbs and index fingers to locate the seminal ducts, which are above the testicles. Roll them around gently, first stretching out to the side, then pulling back, and then stretching forward and out. Use pinching and releasing movements along the length of the ducts as well. Perform each of these actions at least nine times, up to thirty-six times each. Be gentle and careful; the purpose is to massage the ducts so blood will flow more freely through them.

Tapping the Dragon Pearls
Grasp the penis with the right hand directly under the glans penis and stretch it upward. With the middle finger of the left hand, tap gently against each testicle thirty-six times, using enough energy to cause the testicles to bounce up and down. Change the position of the hands and tap each testicle thirty-six times with the right middle finger.

Rolling the Dragon Pearls
Grasp the penis with the right hand, as in the previous exercise. Cup the testicles with the left hand and roll them, using half-twisting motions (much like turning a doorknob), in the hand for a count of thirty-six in each direction. Change hands and repeat the rolling of the testicles with the right hand while stretching the penis with the left hand.

Wearing the Dragon Collar
A Dragon Collar is a silk band that is tied around the base of the penis and scrotum. Before binding, perform the slapping and twisting exercises described previously so that the penis is stimulated.

Don't bind the band too tightly, but just enough to trap blood in the shaft and head of the penis. Wear the collar for at least one hour a day; this will help lengthen the penis and enlarge the head of the penis.

Supplemental Treatments

The following supplemental treatments are used in conjunction with either the Joyful Dragon or Dragon Horn herbal formulas and the Nine Jade Dragon Exercises. These treatments are highly recommended but are not necessary for achieving a larger penis.

Strengthening the Erection

Many men are not able to maintain an erection for a specific amount of time without constant stimulation. Some men find it difficult to attain an erection as quickly as they would like, and some can't keep the erection for as long as they would like. Even men who acquire immediate erections upon stimulation and are able to maintain them would still like to make them stronger. Stronger erections feel good to both the man and his sexual partner.

Aging is also a problem, because the erection becomes diminished in both intensity and duration. Sexual research indicates that after the age of thirty a man fails to attain full erection; the intensity, duration, and frequency of the erection begin to diminish; and the man is less likely to have more than one climax during a single sexual encounter. So it is important to prevent erectile dysfunction before it ever occurs.

The first rule for strengthening erections is to masturbate less frequently. The basic rule is that after the age of thirty, a man should masturbate once a week, at most two to three times. Masturbation desensitizes the penis, especially the *frenum praeputii*, the fold of skin that attaches the underside of the glans penis to the shaft of the penis. Sometimes called the "male clitoris," this skin is very sensitive. After climax it is extremely sensitive, and many men do not like to have it touched for several minutes.

The man who masturbates frequently desensitizes the *frenum praeputii* so that it becomes more and more difficult to maintain an erection if his partner doesn't grasp the penis with the same pressure and apply the same speed and movement as the man performs during masturbation. Another problem is that many men use a lubricant during masturbation, which makes it difficult for them to achieve orgasm or maintain their erections during sex because it does not feel the same as masturbation.

Men can have very intense orgasms as a result of masturbation, and as a result they may not orgasm when with a partner. These problems also occur in women who use vibrators frequently.

There are several simple actions a man can take to strengthen his erections, no matter what type of problem he may be having:

1. Masturbate as often as you like, but only to the point of stimulation, not ejaculation. This will greatly increase your sexual energy as well as strengthen your erections and increase seminal fluid production. It will also help reverse much of the desensitizing that may have occurred.
2. Wear tighter underwear so that more blood remains trapped within the penis during your daily activities.
3. Take either fresh ginger or ginger capsules each day. Ginger has numerous health benefits, one of which is increasing blood circulation to the extremities; this is especially beneficial to the penis and groin.
4. Stimulate what yogis refer to as the kundalini gland. This gland is located a couple of inches inside the anal orifice, and

when stimulated it can greatly strengthen an erection. While lying on your back, have your partner insert the middle finger (with the palm of the hand facing down) fully into your anus, and then press down repeatedly with the finger in the rectum. Have your partner tightly grasp the base of the penis and scrotum with the other index finger and thumb. The effects of the erection will be felt more fully if your partner orally stimulates the glans penis while tapping on the kundalini gland.

Enlarging the Glans Penis

The width of the glans penis is what gives your partner the most pleasure and sensation, whether vaginally, anally, or orally. The glans penis contains the largest majority of the penis's sensory nerves, making it the most sensitive area for the man; for the woman, the rim of the glans penis induces increased sensation within her orifices.

Therefore, the larger the glans penis (the bottom rim especially), the greater the sensation for both partners.

There are three primary methods for enlarging the glans penis. One is to soak the glans penis in warm (not lukewarm or hot) water to increase blood flow. Do this daily for a hundred days, and then stop for thirty days before starting again.

The second method is to have your partner grasp and apply pressure to the base of the penis shaft and entire scrotum with the index finger and thumb of one hand. She should then orally stimulate the head of the penis, using firm suction of her lips and mouth for several seconds; this will also help draw blood into the glans penis. This exercise should be repeated for three to four minutes a day for a hundred days, and then stopped for thirty days before beginning again.

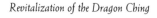

The third method is applying the Dragon Collar directly beneath the glans penis and keeping it there until the erection has subsided. This will help trap blood in the glans penis for a longer period of time, helping to stretch and expand the glans penis.

All of these exercises, along with the Nine Jade Dragon Exercises and the herbal formulas, will greatly help increase the size of the glans penis.

Enhancing Sexual Energy

There are several commonsense actions you can take to ensure that your sexual energy is as high as possible.

- First, maintain some sort of daily exercise routine.
- Second, eat healthy foods, especially vegetables and fruits, and avoid processed foods or those containing sugar. Sugar will only deplete your sexual energy, and over time it completely destroys the energy.
- Third, be hygienic. When the body is clean it is far more energetic. Every day you should apply a cream, lotion, or herbal extract to the entire penis shaft, penis head, and scrotum. Creams containing ginseng, aloe vera, and vitamin E are best, and will help keep the skin smooth and rid the penis shaft of any blemishes or stains.
- Fourth, stay away from cigarettes. Nicotine has been proven to adversely affect blood flow to the penis and can cause impotence. Likewise, limit your coffee consumption; caffeine, like sugar, will deplete your energy. You should absolutely avoid recreational drugs. More than anything else, drugs will, over a

relatively short period of time, cause numerous sexual dysfunctions in a man. Alcohol, if consumed moderately, can increase sexual desire, but if consumed to the point of drunkenness it will dull your senses. It is best to limit yourself to one or two drinks before sex.

Here are some less obvious ways to enhance your sexual energy:

- Shave the entire pubic and groin area. When the genitals are shaved it triggers adolescent responses in the body, making you feel younger and much more energetic. The genitals can also be cleaned more thoroughly and easily, and your partner will take more pleasure in licking the groin and fellating you. It will also help make the penis look younger.
- Have a cup of American ginseng tea twice a day. Never take ginseng when you are sick, however, especially when suffering from a cold, and do not eat white radishes or turnips while consuming ginseng. Ginseng is the highest yang (positive) energy herb there is, it can make a cold virus stronger. White radishes and turnips have extreme yin (negative) energy, and they will create stagnation or poor blood flow in the circulatory system if taken with ginseng. Under the right conditions, taking ginseng twice a day will ensure that a man's sexual and physical energy stay high.
- Each day for sixty days, eat two ounces of crushed walnuts. This will help restore sexual energy, strengthen erections, and increase semen quantity. After sixty days, stop ingesting the walnuts for ninety days and then begin the process again.

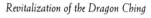

Preventing Nocturnal Emissions

While sitting or lying down, take your right thumbnail and press it into the skin below the center of each fingernail of your left hand. Switch hands and repeat. Press each finger ten times. Do this two times a day. These acupressure points on the fingers calm the kidneys and central nervous system and regulate the seminal ducts.

Preventing Premature Ejaculation

According to the Kinsey reports, the average man ejaculates within four minutes of stimulation. If you sense that your climax is coming too rapidly, apply the following technique to prolong your sexual activity.

While the penis is erect place the index finger and thumb of the left hand around the base of the penis shaft, applying firm pressure with the index finger against the lower part of the underside of the penis. With the index finger and thumb of the right hand squeeze the tip of the penis thirty-six times. Caution must be taken not to pinch the tip of the penis too hard or it might cause bruising. The pressure should be strong enough for you to feel it but light enough not to cause you any pain or discomfort.

Increasing Semen Quantity and Quality

The two parts of a man's sexual performance that will most impress a sexual partner are his intensity at climax and how much semen he ejaculates. The majority of Tigresses claim they love seeing a man ejaculate; they find it intriguing to watch. It also makes them feel good about their sexual performance. The more semen a man ejaculates, the more the woman views herself as having really fulfilled him.

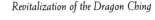

The size of the penis can impress a woman, but even a man with a three-inch penis can excite a woman if he knows how to use his penis well, has a strong erection, has intense orgasms, and ejaculates a lot of semen. The same cannot be said of a man with a large penis that does not function properly, or a man who doesn't properly stimulate his partner.

Aside from the herbs and exercises mentioned previously, the following can also be performed to help the body produce more semen:

- For thirty days soak the scrotum in cold tap water for three minutes. Wait thirty days before performing the soak again. Within a year you should be able to double the amount of semen you normally produce, provided you are also taking the herbs and doing the exercises described earlier in the chapter.
- Take a piece of sliced red ginseng every day and place it in your mouth until it completely dissolves.
- Ejaculate only once in every three masturbations. The other two times, stop before the sensation of climax occurs and simply relax until the urge to climax disappears. This may be hard for some men to do, but repeated ejaculation adversely affects the quantity of semen.
- Let your sexual partner see you ejaculate. Rather than ejaculating inside her or into a condom, do so on her body or on yours. This also might seem difficult, but it will create two important and much-needed psychological responses: first, you will want to ejaculate more semen because you are, in essence, exhibiting it; second, your partner will want to draw more semen from you. Ejaculating more semen will also make

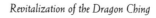

your orgasm more intense and visible for her. Simply put, men love and need to exhibit their virility, and this will psychologically make you want to ejaculate more semen.

- For those who are fond of oral sex, it is advisable to eat either fresh cinnamon, licorice root, or pineapple to make the semen taste better. (Note that ground cinnamon, licorice candy, and processed pineapple juice are not very effective.) Since dairy products and sugar (of which alcohol is primarily based) make the semen taste bitter or rancid, avoid them as much as possible.

Virgin Boy Training

For men who want to completely restore and regenerate their sexual energy and fluids, Virgin Boy Training works best—but it can be difficult. This method was used throughout China in martial arts training and various spiritual practices to ensure that the practitioner's energy would be that of a young boy's again.

The method is easy in theory: Don't have sex or ejaculate for a hundred days. But this is difficult for many men to do. You are advised to practice the acupressure method for preventing nocturnal emissions (see page 83) every day when undertaking this practice. Also, you cannot practice the Nine Jade Dragon Exercises during this time.

The reason for this practice is to restore the semen back to its original healthy and potent condition. If nocturnal emissions do occur, continue practicing but add an extra day to the practice for each nocturnal emission.

At the end of the hundred days you may resume normal sexual activity. However, you will sense how much energy ejaculation takes from you, so you will for a few weeks find yourself refraining from casual masturbation and sex. One of the unfortunate conditions in life is that men are in most instances de-energized by sex while women are frequently energized by it. Men have to be more careful about their frequency of ejaculation, whereas women do not. In fact, the more a woman reaches climax, the healthier it is for her body.

Final Comment

As stated previously, the regimens presented in this chapter are for the purpose of developing strong ching. Some men may wish to practice the methods purely for the purposes of increasing their sexual prowess, penis size, and semen quantity. There is nothing wrong with this, but for the male who wishes to further delve into the more spiritual aspects of Taoist sexuality, these exercises are the foundation for increasing ching and developing the qi and shen. The next three chapters are crucial to the man's sexual-spiritual development.

FOUR

The Sexual Counsel
of the Plain Girl

The following is a *White Tigress Manual* version of the famous Chinese bedchamber text *The Plain Girl Classic (Su Nu Ching)*, which is sometimes referred to as *Counsel of the Plain Girl*. In this *White Tigress Manual* version, the character for sex (hsing) had been inserted into the title, *Hsing Su Nu Ching*, for clarification of the subject matter, I assume. There are several versions of this text in the Chinese language, some of which refer to the benefits a man can acquire from practicing such techniques, and others that detail the benefits for the woman as well. In this version, the male is accentuated, yet there is much knowledge for the female. Also this version is the only one that refrains from exclusive adoption of sexual intercourse. Rather it uses the term *sexual activity* so as to include the beneficial use of oral sex. I cannot prove, however, whether this was added to the text by someone within a past White Tigress lineage or whether it is something that originally appeared in this version. Nonetheless, when comparing this text with other versions, it is apparent that this one is much more eclectic and balanced in its treatment of how a man and woman respect and mutually benefit each other in their sharing of sexual activity and sexual energy.

The Sexual Teachings of the Jade Dragon accomplishes two goals that I felt the companion book, *The Sexual Teachings of the White Tigress*, did not. First, the underlying message, within all sexual situations, is to maintain the utmost respect for the woman's feelings, satisfaction, and comfort. Second, the disciplined control over a man's frequency of ejaculation so as not to injure himself physically or spiritually is why this text is considered so important to the practice of the Jade Dragon—but mostly during the time before and after entering a three-year agreement with a White Tigress.

The text in this chapter is attributed to the Yellow Emperor, Huang Ti, who is believed to have lived from 2697 to 2598 B.C.E., but the first edition of the work did not appear until the Han dynasty, around 225 B.C.E. In the text, Plain Girl answers the Yellow Emperor's questions on sexual matters, and in some cases her counterparts Multihued Girl and Mysterious Girl give their advice. We also find Plain Girl going to seek the advice of Huang Ti's advisor, Feng Tsu, and that of Peng Tsu, who in Chinese mythical legend lived to be more than 800 years old.

Plain Girl, Multihued Girl, and Mysterious Girl were all disciples

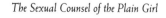

and attendants of the Western Royal Mother (Hsi Wang Mu), who attained immortality through sexual practices. The Yellow Emperor, whose health was failing because of his sexual overindulgence, sought the advice of Plain Girl in order to restore his physical constitution and to receive the necessary knowledge for attaining immortality. But this part of the text primarily focuses on advice for how the Yellow Emperor can restore himself.

The text is presented in five books or sections. The first book, which is called The Tao of Yin-Yang Sexual Harmony, contains four parts and acts as an introduction and overview of the entire book. The second book, which is called Criteria for Developing Sexual Energy, contains six parts and focuses more on the development of sexual energy through the Yellow Emperor's perceptions of women and his conduct while interacting with them. The third book, which is called Methods for Developing Sexual Energy, contains three parts and provides instructions for techniques meant to enhance a man's sexual energy. The fourth book, which is called Perceiving the Signs of Female Sensuality, contains four parts and is a guide that describes how men might better read the sexual desires and needs of females. The fifth book, which is called Sexual Postures, Techniques, and Therapies, contains five parts and is a very broad section dealing with the most healthy and yin-yang balanced procedures for sex.

The main premise of this text is how to balance the yin and yang aspects during the sex act, and it strongly advocates infrequent ejaculation for the man and frequent orgasm for the woman. Therefore, it is upon this premise that the Jade Dragon finds this work so invaluable in his quest for health, longevity, and immortality.

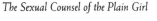

Introduction to the Plain Girl Classic

The Yellow Emperor, sensing his mortality, requested the counsel of the immortaless, Mysterious Girl: "It is known to me that there were people of ancient times who lived to well over a hundred years of age, yet remained in perfect health and as active as if in their twenties. Presently it seems that people only reach half that age before their health fails and the body becomes decrepit. Is the reason for this because each passing generation degenerates itself? Or is it that we have neglected or forgotten some secret law of nature?"

The Mysterious Girl responded: "These ancient people lived according to the natural workings of Yin and Yang, and cultivated the arts of joyful bliss between man and woman. They did not care about living one hundred years or more, rather living each moment in joy was their Tao. How can there be joy in life if one is constantly engaged in striving to live one hundred years or more? They lived and cherished each moment of joyful bliss and so acquired longevity without striving. Thoughts of death, aging, and illness never occurred to them.

"In eating and drinking they were moderate; their periods of activity and rest were regular; and were never disorderly or prone to excessive behaviors. Without prejudice or ill emotions they compassionately enjoined in joyful bliss for the betterment of

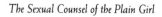

harmony between the sexes. Living tranquilly and harmoniously was their natural temperament. It was then by these measures that they could live one hundred years or more in perfect health.

"But presently people are not like this; their eating, drinking, activities, periods of rest, and behaviors are all treated recklessly. When they enter the bedchamber they exhaust their vital forces (*qi*); dissipate their true essence (*ching*); and cannot control or focus their spirit (*shen*). Wishing only to selfishly amuse and benefit themselves, they cannot find true contentment within, and so cut themselves off from long-life and joyful bliss.

"In ancient times people followed the teachings of the immortalesses and immortals; they were tranquil and content in abiding in nothingness; always maintaining their vital forces; their original spirit was preserved internally so no illness could affect them. They had no selfish desires, so their hearts were at peace and without fear, even though they applied themselves wholeheartedly to every task they never felt wearied. With their spirits in harmony and obedience, everything was satisfactory to them and all they wished for could be achieved. They were happy under any conditions, and were unconcerned whether another person was of high or low position in life; whether they were beautiful or mediocre in appearance; whether they were coarse or refined in temperament; whether they were aggressive or passive in nature. These people were pure of heart because they did not discriminate against others; they were nonjudgmental toward others; and they did not interfere with others. They recognized the beauty and potential for joyful bliss in everyone around them, always living

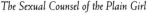

in accordance with the natural laws of yin and yang replenishing each other. These people lived the true Tao because they understood and emulated Heaven's creativity and the earth's receptivity, thereby living in full humanity."

The Yellow Emperor asked, "When people grow old they can no longer give birth to children or enter the bedchamber to experience joyful bliss. Is this because they exhausted their regenerative essences during youth, or is it just a natural fate of everyone?"

The Mysterious Girl responded, "Listen carefully, the secret methods of the ancients regarding restoration and long life according to the natural laws of yin and yang will be imparted to you, which were all transmitted to me by the Western Royal Mother (Hsi Wang Mu)."

Secrets of Longevity for Females

"When a girl is seven years of age, the qi in her ovaries and kidneys is quite abundant, her teeth undergo change, and her hair begins to grow longer. Physically active and strong her saliva flows abundantly. Her Jade Gate is unbroken and so her ching has not been dissipated or injured. Her yin and yang are in harmony and needs no absorption or replenishment from yang essences.

"When she turns fourteen she has begun to menstruate regularly and can give birth to a child. The movement of qi within the two meridians, *jen* and *mo*, is strong, causing her hips to widen, her breasts to swell, her sexual curiosity peaks and so begins to seek the attention of males. If her Jade Gate is broken she will begin aging; if unbroken she can preserve her youthfulness for a few

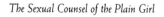

more years. Her yang forces are just beginning to wane and so she seeks to replenish them.

"When she reaches the age of twenty-one the qi of her kidneys remains level, her adult teeth are in place, and she is a full-grown woman, requiring the amorous attention of males and release of her Jade Gate secretions to preserve her health and youthfulness. Once the Jade Gate secretions are released, she will need to begin replenishing herself through absorption of yang forces.

"When she reaches the age of twenty-eight her muscles and bones are strong, her hair reaches its full length, and her body is physically strong and fertile. She more frequently needs release of her Jade Gate secretions. However, if her Jade Gate remains unbroken she will now begin aging more rapidly because her yin begins to stagnate and wane, she will need to absorb yang essences in order to replenish her waning yin essences.

"When she reaches the age of thirty-five the qi within the pulses of the stomach (*yang ming*, sunlight) begin deteriorating, her breasts begin to sag, her face shows signs of wrinkling, and she begins losing hair. Because the qi within her stomach wanes, she needs more frequent release of secretions, but less invasion of her Jade Gate in order to maintain youthfulness. She will now more frequently need to absorb yang essences in order to maintain youthful vigor.

"When she reaches the age of forty-two the qi in the pulses in the upper three yang regions of her body begin to deteriorate, especially affecting the breasts, throat, and eyes. Her face becomes ever more wrinkled and her hair begins turning white. In order to deflect the effects of the waning three yang regions, she needs to produce more saliva and Jade Gate secretions, as well as absorb increased amounts of yang essence.

"When she reaches the age of forty-nine she can no longer be impregnated and the circulation of qi through the *jen* and *mo* meridians decreases. Her menstrual cycle is exhausted and the secretions of her Jade Gate wane. In order to prevent old age from permanently setting in she needs very frequent simulation of her Jade Gate secretions, increased production of saliva, and frequent absorption of yang essences.

"Your majesty, can you now understand the process by which a female either ages or retains her youthfulness? Is it not clear that a female suffers from rapid aging because of seven traumas:

1. Breaking of the Jade Gate before age twenty-eight; not breaking the Jade Gate after age twenty-eight.
2. Too frequent activity of intercourse.
3. Lack of frequent release and production of the Jade Gate secretions.
4. Lack of adequate saliva production.
5. Not maintaining the flow of qi in *jen* and *mo* meridians.
6. Not maintaining the flow of qi in the stomach and three yang regions.
7. Not absorbing frequently enough the yang essences of males to replenish their yin.

"By avoiding these seven traumas a female can restore and pre-serve her youthfulness well beyond the age of forty-nine, as well as open the door for acquiring the secrets of longevity and immortality."

Secrets of Longevity for Males

"When a boy is eight years of age, the qi in his testes and kidneys is quite abundant, his teeth undergo change, and his hair begins to grow longer. Physically active and strong his saliva flows abundantly. His Jade Stem experiences frequent erections, but his ching has not been dissipated or injured. His yin and yang are in harmony and he needs no replenishment from yin essences to maintain that harmony.

"When he turns sixteen the qi of his testes are fully developed and he secretes semen. Having begun to masturbate regularly, he can impregnate a woman. The movement of qi within the two meridians, *jen* and *mo*, is strong, causing his chest and shoulders to expand, and causing an abundance of semen. His sexual appetite begins developing and he seeks the attention of females. If his Jade Stem is used too often he will begin aging; if used moderately he can preserve his youthfulness for a few more years. His yin forces are beginning to wane and so he seeks to replenish them.

"When he reaches the age of twenty-four the qi of his testes and kidneys remains level, his adult teeth are in place, muscles and bones are firm and strong, and having reached his full height, he is now a fully grown man. He requires the amorous attention of females and release of his semen to preserve his health and youthfulness, otherwise it can cause damage and stagnation to the kidneys and testes. But if there is frequent release of his semen, he will need to begin replenishing himself through yin essences.

"When he reaches the age of thirty-two his muscles and bones are strong, his hair reaches its full length, and his body is physically strong and fertile. He more frequently needs release of his semen, but its quantity is beginning to diminish as is the intensity and frequency of his erections. However, if his Jade Stem remains unused he will now begin aging more rapidly because his yang begins to stagnate and wane, he will need to absorb yin essences in order to replenish his waning yang essences.

"When he reaches the age of forty the qi within the testes and kidneys begin deteriorating, his muscles begin to sag, his face shows signs of wrinkling, and he begins losing hair. Because the qi within his testes wanes, he needs less frequent release of semen but more contact with females in order to maintain youthfulness. He will now more frequently need to replenish the yin essences in order to maintain youthful vigor.

"When he reaches the age of forty-eight the qi in the pulses in the lower three yang regions of his body begin to deteriorate, especially affecting the testes, kidneys, and Jade Stem. His face becomes ever more wrinkled and his hair begins turning white at the temples. In order to deflect the effects of the waning three yang regions, he needs to produce more saliva, as well as replenish himself with increased amounts of yin essence.

"When he reaches the age of fifty-six the energy of his liver deteriorates and the muscles no longer function properly. The circulation of qi through the *jen* and *mo* meridians decreases. His semen is becoming exhausted and the frequency of erections wanes. In order to prevent old age from permanently setting in he needs very infrequent dissipation of semen, increased production of saliva, and frequent absorption of yin essences.

"At age sixty-four he begins losing his teeth and hair. He will need to completely prevent all ejaculation and entirely focus on accumulating qi in his abdomen to preserve his health.

"Your majesty, can you now understand the process by which a male either ages or retains his youthfulness? Is it not clear that a male also suffers from rapid aging because of seven traumas:

1. Overuse of the Jade Stem before age twenty-four; not using the Jade Stem after the age twenty-four.
2. Too frequent dissipation of semen.
3. Lack of frequent erections.
4. Lack of adequate saliva production.
5. Not maintaining the flow of qi in *jen* and *mo* meridians.
6. Not maintaining the flow of qi in the stomach and three yang regions.
7. Not absorbing frequently enough the yin essences of females to replenish his yang.

"By avoiding these seven traumas a male can restore and preserve his youthfulness well beyond the age of forty-eight, as well as open the door for acquiring the secrets of longevity and immortality."

The Yellow Emperor then said to Mysterious Girl, "But there are people who already old in years who can produce offspring. There are also those who remain youthful looking and active even though in their senior years. How is all this possible?"

Mysterious Girl smiled and said, "Within the seven traumas for both the male and female lies the opening secrets for preserving youthfulness and attaining immortality. The ancients knew the workings of nature, imitated it and so could live over a hundred years in perfect health and contentment. Your majesty, deteriorating condition is a result of not working with the yin and yang forces of nature."

Mysterious Girl then rose to the sky and beckoned for Plain Girl to come and impart to the Yellow Emperor the secrets of yin and yang harmony that all men should know.

BOOK I
The Tao of Yin-Yang Sexual Harmony
The Sexual Joys of Regulating Yin and Yang

The Yellow Emperor asked of Plain Girl, "My entire body and mind feels exhausted and in disharmony. Constantly I feel an anxiety about being on the verge of some coming peril and that my days are coming to and end. What is causing this?"

Plain Girl responded, "This is due to an overall imbalance of your yin and yang, because you have obviously been careless with your sex life. You have obviously been involved with women whose sexuality and sexual desire were much stronger than yours, and you have been unable to maintain adequate sexual stamina to ward off their energy. This is not unlike a fire being put out by water. Sexual activity between a man and a woman is akin to the proper regulation of fire and water when cooking, so that delicious and hot food can be made. Therefore, the regulation of fire and water must be paid close attention so that the sexual energy and pleasure can be gathered and enjoyed to the utmost extent. Without this regulation the physical body will break down and death will come much more quickly. How then can you enjoy your life? You have to learn to be much more aware of how you conduct yourself sexually."

Plain Girl then added, "I know a woman, her name is Multi-hued Girl, and she is very wise about the workings of yin and yang." The Yellow Emperor asked Plain Girl to go see Multihued Girl and learn from her the secrets for attaining longevity and how to maintain a proper balance within his sex life.

Feng Tsu, listening to this conversation, told Plain Girl, "If a man treats his sexual energy (ching) as a treasure through meditation and the ingesting of the correct herbal medicines, he can achieve a long life and spiritual immortality. However, if a man does not learn the correct principles of regulating his sexual energy, then no matter how much he may practice nourishing regimens or ingest herbal medicines, it will do him no good.

"The sexual behaviors and activities between a man and

woman are identical to how the universe itself came into creation. Like Heaven and Earth, the male and female share a parallel relationship in attaining an immortal existence. They both must learn how to engage and develop their natural sexual instincts and behaviors; otherwise the only result is decay and traumatic discord of their physical lives. However, if they engage in the utmost joys of sensuality and apply the principles of yin and yang to their sexual activity, their health, vigor, and joy of love will bear them the fruits of longevity and immortality."

The Tao of Loving and Sensuality

The Yellow Emperor commented to Mysterious Girl, "I have understood the basic concepts for regulating the yin and yang from Plain Girl. But I now pray you will explain the inner secrets and details of this."

Mysterious Girl responded, "There is nothing within Heaven and Earth that is not created through the intermingling of yin and yang. The birth of an infant begins when yang interacts with yin, and the maturity of the individual takes place because the yin nourishes itself with the yang. The harmonious coexistence of both yin and yang within an individual is greatly affected by how they are balanced and maintained. An individual's existence is either benefited or injured by this balance and maintenance of yin and yang.

"Therefore, when a man brings his penis into contact with a woman, an erection occurs. When a woman becomes sexually

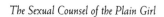

stimulated, her labia open. So when these two elements of yang and yin appear, the man's semen is produced and the female's secretions begin to flow and the harmonious union of male and female—yin and yang—sexual energy begins to culminate.

"Within sexual interaction the male must follow the principles of the Eight Sexual Rules and the woman must adhere to the Nine Sexual Rules. Both the male and female must abide by their respective rules, otherwise the man could experience painful swelling of the joints and various ulcers and the woman could experience amenorrhea or other illnesses. Not adhering to the rules over a long period of time will result in an early death. By adhering to the rules of properly balancing and maintaining the sexual energies these principles of yin and yang will bring to each partner health, happiness, and longevity."

A Moment of Bliss is Worth a Thousand Gold Pieces

The Yellow Emperor went on to ask for further instruction on and definition of the principles of yin and yang in regard to sexual activity.

Plain Girl replied, "Sex between males and females is a natural act that determines and produces a higher quality of life. If sexual activity is practiced in accordance with the principles of yin and yang, the male will greatly enhance both his prowess and energy and the female can eradicate illnesses and restore her youthfulness. Both the male and female can experience inner joy, live in good health, and be full of enlivened spirit. However, if they do not maintain the principles of yin and yang within their sexual activity, their bodies will suffer imbalances and be hastened toward deterioration.

"To answer your question about the principles of yin and yang in regard to sexual activity, I say this: There must be mental discipline, harmonizing of the internal energy, emotional balance, and both bodily and intellectual congruence. Never expose yourself to extremes; keep yourself from extreme cold and heat, never eat too much and never too little, never be fanatical about ethics and morality, and always seek to be naturally at peace with yourself and others.

"Sexual activity is never to be considered as an end in itself, as it is but part of a larger scheme designed to develop love and the natural exchange of male and female sexual energies. All sexual activity should be embarked on first with mutual respect, love, and great anticipation.

"If sexual activity is to have spiritual significance and if the yin and yang are to be properly enjoined, then each partner must have the proper attitude and feeling to fully experience the activity. It is for this reason that sexual activity must be undertaken with an attitude of harmony and gentleness. Approach everything slowly and with awareness of what is taking place. Make a concerted effort to feel and sense the actuality of the other person's energy and sensation.

"After this period of feeling and sensing sexual activity should then take place. The man may place his Jade Stem (penis) near the woman's Red Lotus (tongue) and Jade Chamber (vagina), but

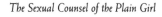

he must do so gently and slowly. All violent or hard movements must be avoided if the heights of pleasure and joy are to be attained."

Tranquillity and Natural Elation

The Yellow Emperor then inquired, "I wanted to engage in sexual activity, but my Jade Stem would not become erect. During this I felt great shame as I stood there drenched in my own sweat in front of this young woman, feeling that I had no place in which to hide myself.

"Eventually I managed to insert my Jade Stem inside her Jade Chamber, yet to no avail. How could I have maintained the correct physical response? Please be kind enough to tell me the secret details of this."

The Plain Girl answered him: "The emperor's problem is common to many men. Now, when a man seeks to have sexual activity with a woman he should always prepare himself mentally by approaching it slowly and in a progressive manner. But the most important thing is to calm the mind; once that occurs the Jade Stem will stand and remain erect.

"The man must also observe the Five Empowerments: kindness, proper conduct, manners, knowledge, and sincerity. Along with these he must know how to properly stimulate her Nine Erogenous Areas. Then, when expressing his sexual desire for her, he will be able to show his full appreciation for her Five Beautiful Qualities and so benefit from the union. With all these, a new stamina and vigor will fill his entire body.

"Initially a man should kiss the lips of a woman and gather into his mouth her saliva, which will help him build his stamina and will imbue his brain with sexual energy. Through this he can also ward off the injuries caused by the Seven Traumas. Then, applying the techniques of the Eight Benefits, he will not contradict his adherence to the Five Empowerments. It is in this manner that a man can achieve optimum health and build his stamina and vigor. He will never have to worry about mental or physical diseases encroaching on him."

Plain Girl then added, "When a man's internal organs and bowels are properly functioning and fit, his countenance will be glowing and healthy. When engaged in sexual activity his Jade Stem will become as erect as an iron bar, and thus he will fully enjoy the sexual activity as long he wishes. If a man adheres to the Five Empowerments, he will not suffer from impotence."

BOOK II
Criteria for Developing Sexual Energy

Qi

The Yellow Emperor asked of Plain Girl, "I have been considering not having sexual activity for awhile. What is your opinion of this?"

Plain Girl said, "You cannot do it. The two aspects of Heaven and Earth [yin and yang] are in constant flux between opening

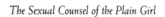

and closing, and are always at variance with one another. This is not unlike the changes of the four seasons of spring, summer, autumn, and winter, or that of day and night with the constant flux of lightness and darkness. All these changes are what maintain human life. So to human beings must abide by the natural variances of yin and yang, just as they must act in accordance with the changing of the four seasons.

"When a person suppresses and stops sexual activity, the energy and vitality can not then be vented, and the intermingling of yin and yang is obstructed. If this happens it is then impossible to keep the tone of the physical body, which is normally provided through sexual activity. It is absolutely necessary that the qi of the body be allowed to move so that it may aid in the venting of waste gasses and other injurious elements of the body. Therefore, learning the proper methods of breathing during sexual activity can greatly benefit your health.

"Your Majesty, it is said in the *Secrets of the Jade Chamber* that a man should put forth great effort in expanding his abdomen with his breath during sexual activity so that he may increase his physical strength and stamina. So when the woman is stimulating his Jade Stem with either her Red Lotus or Jade Gate, he is to take a deep breath, hold it for a count of thirty, and then exhale. He should repeat this several times. This will ensure he maintains a hard erection.

"Also, immediately upon sensing his ejaculation he should grasp his Jade Stem and remove it from her stimulation, and after the erection has softened somewhat, he should bring it back to her for stimulation again. This is done repeatedly. Over a ten-day period of practicing this, the Jade Stem will become like hardened steel and hot as a flaming torch. This will ensure greater and prolonged sexual activity."

The Setting

The Yellow Emperor again asked of Plain Girl, "What is the ideal criteria for conducting sexual activity between a man and woman?"

Plain Girl answered, "The foundation of ideal sexual activity lies in both the person's nature and his sexual instincts. With natural sexual activity [procreation] aside, males and females both need to learn the principles of yin and yang and the appropriate sexual techniques in order to bear the fruits of their sexuality and activities.

"Now, if they understand and master these principles and techniques they will gain healthy bodies, increased mental capacities, and endless vigor. But if the Tao of these principles is not followed, weakness and dullness will ensue. Indeed, the most important factors leading to the joys of sexual activity are in balanced emotions, mental relaxation, and a strong spirit. If these three factors are achieved, both the male and female will greatly increase their stamina and vigor. Simultaneously, all illnesses, physical or mental, that might encroach upon them will be naturally resisted.

"During all sexual activity, especially during the initial contact, the man must never attempt to just thrust or force his Jade Stem into the woman's Jade Gate or on the Red Lotus. Rather, he must move slowly and gently, allowing her to feel the pleasures and sensations of the activity. This will allow him to maintain his physical and sexual health."

Plain Girl then broke into song,

> *There must be a sense of security between them, so their*
>   *hearts are tranquil.*
> *There must be a harmony of minds between them, so*
>   *there will be no conflict.*
> *The chamber must not be too cold or too warm,*
>   *and their stomachs neither too full nor too empty.*
> *Stopping only when she is completely satisfied and*
>   *when he is not yet exhausted.*

The Need for Loving Touch

The Yellow Emperor asked Mysterious Girl, "Please instruct me as to what to do about a female who during sexual foreplay becomes frigid and exhibits no desire for sexual activity, and her vagina does not moisten. In men, sometimes the Jade Stem will become erect, but then will shrink and become flaccid. What are the reasons for this?"

Mysterious Girl responded, "The aspects of yin and yang need to be balanced to be effective in sexual activity. Therefore, when the man's yang aspects [male stimulation of the female] are properly stimulated, the female is enabled to give and receive sexual pleasure. Likewise, the man must be aroused by the yin aspects [female stimulation of the male], otherwise he cannot achieve and maintain an erection. In this situation, if the male insists on having sex, the female will be uncomfortable. Contrarily, if the female insists on union, the man will lack vigor and stamina.

"Now, if both the female and male have mutual desire and affection for each other, they are harmonious and will stimulate each other, and so be able to enjoy both the giving and receiving of their sexual activity. On the other hand, if they are of different minds, and one of them is without the intent to stimulate, the fire for stimulation will be extinguished. No matter what, if sexual activity is being forced by either one, only rejection will ensue from the other.

"When the Jade Stem secretes Dragon Rain and the man presses this slowly and gently on the woman's chin, breasts, or vagina it will cause her to become excited. The male can then advance the activity, as she will begin stimulating him in whatever manner and at whatever speed he requests. The female will then naturally respond to the movements of the Jade Stem and will open and contract the orifice [mouth or vagina] being stimulated. In this manner the male will not have to exert too much energy in order to stimulate and please the female, allowing everything to happen naturally instead.

"At this time the male can absorb the yin energy of the female and increase his physical strength. He does so by adhering to and perfecting the Eight Sensual Techniques: opening, closing, lying

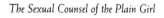

on the stomach, lying on the back, withdrawing thrusts, advancing thrusts, circling, and bending. The male should always be in accord with these eight techniques during sexual activity."

Rules for Sexual Activity

The Yellow Emperor then asked Plain Girl, "Concerning the sexual conduct between a male and female, is there any specific order in which these behaviors should be observed?"

Plain Girl responded, "Yes. First the female is to lie back in a comfortable position with her legs apart. The male then kneels between her legs and stimulates her vagina with delicate kissing and brisk tongue movements over this entire area. The man should then take his Jade Stem and press it gently around the labia and especially on the clitoris. When the woman is fully stimulated they may begin the sexual activity of their choosing.

"The insertion of the Jade Stem, be it vaginal or oral, must follow in accordance with the Eight Sensual Techniques and it should be performed gradually according to the depth. Each depth is to be enjoyed fully before moving on to the next depth. This is the orderly rule for sexual activity."

The Yellow Emperor said, "During sexual activity you say that the male must know how to control the depth of insertion properly or neither the male nor female will fully enjoy or receive the benefits of sexual pleasure. Please tell me in detail how to properly control the depth of insertion of the Jade Stem."

Plain Girl answered, "A male must always be conscious and

sensitive to what the female's sexual needs are and he must satisfy them, all the while treasuring his ching and never ejaculating his semen haphazardly. First he should rub his hands together vigorously to make them warm. He should then hold the base of his Jade Stem firmly and place it either against the female's labia or within the opening of her mouth. In either case he should move the Jade Stem back and forth somewhat briskly. After the female is well moistened and secretions ooze from her vagina or saliva spills from her mouth, he should alternately use shallow insertion followed by a somewhat deeper insertion of the Jade Stem. If the male can maintain this motion, he will heighten the stimulation of the female and give her more self-confidence about her ability to give and receive pleasure.

"The insertion of the Jade Stem must not be too fast or too slow; the important part is to not forcefully thrust the Jade Stem too deeply, which might cause injury or pain to the woman. The male should begin with several insertions at a depth of one inch and then alternate these with a deeper insertion of two inches. When she reaches a state of heightened mental intensity she will unconsciously tighten her facial muscles and perspire and her breath will quicken, her eyes will shut, and her face will feel hot. Her vagina will likewise open and begin to flow with secretions, her cheeks will redden, and her mouth will flow with saliva. The male should be aware of these effects, as it means her mind and body are replenishing the yang with the yin and she is experiencing great pleasure.

"Your Majesty, you should also become knowledgeable about the Eight Valleys within a woman: the Lute String Valley, at a depth of one inch; the Water Chestnut Valley, at a depth of two inches; the Little Brook Valley, at a depth of three inches; the Black Pearl Valley, at a depth of four inches; the Simple Valley, at a depth of five inches; the Dark Chamber Valley, at a depth of six inches; the Inner Gate Valley, at a depth of seven inches; and the Pole Star Valley, at a depth of eight inches."

The Five Constant Virtues

The Yellow Emperor asked of Plain Girl, "You mentioned that the orderly rules for sexual activity were based on the Five Constant Virtues. Please tell me what these are?"

Plain Girl responded, "These are the five virtuous uses of the Jade Stem. I will explain each one for you.

"The first of the Five Constant Virtues is when a man who is in seclusion and behaving like a hermit treats his Jade Stem in a benevolent manner by allowing it to remain flaccid, so maintaining celibacy.

"The second of the Five Constant Virtues is when a man never puts forth effort for pleasuring his Jade Stem and as such is considered righteous, only allowing sexual activity to occur if a female asks it of him.

"The third of the Five Constant Virtues is when a man often touches his Jade Stem like he would the end of a rope, but never does so in the presence of a female. As such, he is considered ethical.

"The fourth of the Five Constant Virtues is when a man desires sexual activity and his Jade Stem becomes erect from visualizing women. Yet he is self-composed and nonaggressive, and as such is considered trustworthy and controlled.

"The fifth of the Five Constant Virtues is when a man engaged in sexual activity is in accord with the orderly rules; as such he is considered principled and wise.

"Every man should pay attention to these Five Constant Virtues so he may be able to control his sexual desires and not harm himself with excessive dissipation or violent aggression.

"A male may desire sexual activity even though his energy is not sufficient because he lacks both quality semen and physical stamina. If so he should consider adopting one of the Five Constant Virtues. In doing so he can avoid many physical problems and prevent himself from engaging in excessive sexual activity. By doing this he becomes self-controlled.

"But if a man is ready for sexual activity with a female, he must treat her with sincerity and respect. By doing so, trust and faith will become part and parcel of his relationships and reputation. This will be a testament to his understanding of proper sexual activity."

BOOK III
The Methods for Developing Sexual Energy

The Ebb and Flow of Sexual Energy

Plain Girl questioned Peng Tsu. "What type of symptoms can be seen and recognized concerning the ebb and flow of sexual energy associated in men?" she asked.

Peng Tsu replied, "If the male is in good spirits and feels strong, his Jade Stem will feel hot and the semen will thicken. If sexual desire is waning, these five symptoms will appear: he may ejaculate a scant amount of semen, meaning his mind is full of anxiety; he may ejaculate watery semen, meaning he is undergoing physical stress; he may ejaculate foul-smelling semen, meaning his muscles and tendons have been traumatized; he may ejaculate semen in a dribbling fashion, rather than a forceful spurting of semen, meaning there is a trauma occurring in his bones and joints; he may fail to become erect, meaning that both a physical and psychological trauma are occurring simultaneously.

"These symptoms are usually the result of having been in opposition to the principles of yin and yang, and likely with an accompanying emotional problem. The cure for these problems is to engage in sexual activity without allowing ejaculation. By doing so, within a hundred days the man's stamina and virility will be strengthened a hundredfold."

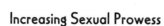

Increasing Sexual Prowess

The Yellow Emperor asked Plain Girl, "Sexual activity usually results in ejaculation. So if I can control my orgasms and prevent my ejaculations, what will be the benefits of this? Please advise me in detail."

Plain Girl said, "Upon the first sensation of ejaculation, if you control it correctly, you will strengthen yourself and enhance your virility. Here are the benefits of restraining ejaculations:

"Restraining the second ejaculation will clear the ears and eyes.

"Restraining the third ejaculation will rid the joints and muscles of the body of soreness and ailments.

"Restraining the fourth ejaculation will strengthen the five internal organs.

"Restraining the fifth ejaculation will regulate all the pulses of the body.

"Restraining the sixth ejaculation will strengthen the spine and waist.

"Restraining the seventh ejaculation will strengthen the buttocks and thighs.

"Restraining the eighth ejaculation will bring youthful color to the skin and a smooth, robust complexion.

"Restraining the ninth ejaculation will naturally increase longevity.

"Restraining the tenth ejaculation will lead you to immortality."

Multihued Girl interjected, saying, "It is normally considered that a man derives utmost pleasure from the sensations of ejaculation.

However, in learning to attain the Tao he is encouraged to ejaculate less and less. In doing so will not his sensation of pleasure also be diminished?"

Peng Tsu responded, "Very far from it. After a man has ejaculated he becomes tired, his ears buzz, and his eyes grow heavy with sleep. He also experiences thirst and his limbs and joints ache and stiffen. When a man ejaculates he experiences pleasure for but a few moments, but suffers weariness for many hours afterwards. How is this true pleasure?"

The Yellow Emperor then asked, "Then how does a man properly prevent ejaculation?"

Plain Girl answered him, "Upon first sensing that you are about to ejaculate stop all movement of the Jade Stem and forcefully press on your pubic area around the base of the Jade Stem with both hands. Breathe in deeply and quickly, then exhale gradually and slowly. Simultaneously grit the teeth together and breathe in slowly and deeply. As you are doing this raise your head to gaze upward and then downward, and then from left to right. Then contract the lower abdomen and relax momentarily.

"Next fill the abdomen and lungs with air so they expand, focusing on your *tan t'ien* while exhaling and contracting your abdomen. Simultaneously gaze upward and relax momentarily. Then breathe in deeply; slowly exhale. Rotate your eyes clockwise three times while contracting the abdomen. Inhale deeply while gritting the teeth together and relax the entire body. When you sense a windlike movement in your ears, contract the abdomen.

"When the erection starts to subside, your breathing and heart will quiet and you will feel in control of your spirit. At this point sexual activity may again be resumed."

The Yellow Emperor asked, "This all seems very good, but is not ejaculation necessary for the purpose of posterity?"

Plain Girl responded, "Each man is different, depending on both his age and his constitution. Every man desires to experience sexual pleasure according to his sexual abilities. However, excessive sexual indulgence will only serve to injure his health and diminish his sense of sexual joy and sensation. To avoid these problems follow these guidelines:

"At age fifteen, if strong and full of vigor, you may ejaculate twice a day. But if you are lacking strength and vigor, and are of slight build, you may ejaculate once a day without causing any ill effects.

"A vigorous twenty year old may ejaculate twice a day. But if he is less vigorous ejaculating once a day is sufficient.

"A vibrant thirty year old may engage in sexual activity leading to ejaculation once per day. But if he is less vibrant once every other day will suffice.

"The lustful forty year old may engage in sexual activity leading to ejaculation once every three days. But the less lustful man should only ejaculate once every four days.

"The virile fifty year old may enjoy sexual activity leading to ejaculation every five days; the less virile, once every ten days.

"A strong seventy year old may enjoy sexual activity leading to ejaculation once every thirty days, but a weak seventy year old is advised not to ejaculate."

Frequent Sexual Activity, Infrequent Ejaculation

Plain Girl continued to query Peng Tsu on his knowledge of these matters. Peng Tsu responded, "The practice of frequent sexual activity and infrequent ejaculation is easy and logical to those who have been properly taught. But the common person does not have the confidence, tenacity, and understanding for the disciplined practice of it.

"Now, the Yellow Emperor is engaged full-time with affairs of his empire, which cause him to be physically and mentally fatigued. All these heavy burdens prevent him from being able to put into practice the principles of yin and yang within his sexual activity.

"The Yellow Emperor is fortunate in that he has many concubines, and if he could only adhere to these methods he could greatly benefit his health, stamina, and virility. Sexual vitality can be greatly increased through frequent sexual activity with young women, provided ejaculation is not frequent. If he could lessen his ejaculation of semen, he would begin to feel light and at ease, and no illness would encroach upon him."

Nine Shallow and One Deep

In counseling the Yellow Emperor, Plain Girl said, "During sexual activity [intercourse] with a woman, the man should regard her as he would a piece of stone, yet regard himself as gold and jade. Should the woman begin to intensely enjoy the pleasure from the sensations and begin to move her body rhythmically and with extreme passion, he must quickly withdraw his Jade Stem from her Jade Gate because she will cause him to ejaculate.

"If it is the case that the man wishes to make the young woman orgasm, the time spent engaged in intercourse must be given cautious attention. This is because attempting to regulate the sexual technique while simultaneously bringing her to orgasm is akin to trying to control a galloping horse while holding a rotted bridle, or standing on the edge of an abyss that is filled below with sharp glistening swords. Therefore, attempting to cause an orgasm for the female during intercourse must be exercised with great caution, because your ejaculation will result in loss of energy and power. So with great effort avoid ejaculation of semen while the female is in the state of orgasm, so that your vitality can be preserved to the utmost.

"According to our ancient ancestors, sexual behaviors and techniques performed by the male in order to seduce a female should begin with gentle caresses. He should begin by lightly touching her fingertips with his hands and then slowly proceed up the arms to her shoulders. Then he should gently touch the tips of her toes and gradually work his way up her thighs until he reaches her mound of Venus.

"All sensual hand caresses should begin with the middle finger, and then gradually add the forefinger and then the ring finger. Ideally all three fingers will come into play to slowly and rhythmically stroke and fondle the woman. Gently stroke the back of her hands, and then the center of her palms. Continue this type of caressing using various circular patterns. Then, after a period of time, move upward along the inner sides of her arms and up to the shoulders.

"After the man finishes caressing the hands and feet, he should bring his left hand around to her backside and draw her closer to him in a gentle hug. The right hand gently strokes her stomach and abdomen and slowly moves down to her mound of Venus.

"Simultaneously with this caressing described, the man should kiss the woman in a methodical manner: first the neck, then the forehead, using both the lips and tongue. He should then proceed to kiss and lick her lips, throat, and breasts, and then he should nibble on her earlobes. With passion he should lick and kiss all the sexually sensitive areas of her body—the abdomen, lower back, buttocks, inner thighs, and genital area. Ideally, he should lick and kiss every part of her body.

"When all the caressing, licking, and kissing is complete she will be sexually responsive and they will be ready for sexual activity. It is important, however, that the man adhere to the techniques of Nine Shallow and One Deep or Eight Shallow and Two Deep. Doing so will ensure her sexual satisfaction."

Plain Girl continued, "During sexual activity the male should in a slow repetitive manner insert the Jade Stem [either nine times shallow and one time deep or eight times shallow and two times deep]. During the shallow movements, the Jade Stem should be directed a little to the left three times and then a little to the right three times. The Jade Stem sways deliberately in this manner, like the movement of a snake or fish. After every ten movements, the Jade Stem is inserted another inch deeper, until finally it is fully inserted.

"The man should perform each deep insertion in coordination with his breathing, inhaling deeply while inserting and withdrawing on the exhale. Shallow insertions are made to the depth between the Lute String Valley and the Black Pearl Valley. Deep insertions are made to the depth between the Little Brook Valley and the Simple Valley. If the man inserts the Jade Stem too shallowly, neither partner will derive the optimum pleasure from their activity; if he inserts it too deeply, she may be injured.

"The Jade Stem should be inserted shallowly nine [or eight] times, so as to bring the female to a state of intense passion, in which she loses all control and restraint. Then the Jade Stem should be fully inserted in one [or two] gentle penetrating thrust[s]. This is the ancient technique called Nine Shallow and One Deep."

BOOK IV
Recognizing the Signs of Female Sensuality
The Nine Energies of the Female

The Yellow Emperor said to Plain Girl, "My understanding of the Four Cardinal Points in regards to a man is sufficient. But what are the Nine Energies of the female?"

Plain Girl responded, "These Nine Energies are not difficult to perceive or understand. They are:

"When the female has the propensity for and is observed breathing hastily, salivating, and swallowing. This means the qi of the lung is abundant.

"When the female has the propensity for and is observed moaning gently when kissing a man, this means the qi of the heart is full.

"When the female has the propensity for and is observed embracing men with both her arms, this means the qi of the spleen is plentiful.

"When the female has the propensity for and is observed with a moist vagina, this means the qi of the kidney is diffusive.

"When the female has the propensity for and is observed flirting with men, and she loves to sensually nibble on their bodies, this means the qi has penetrated the bones and heated the marrow.

"When the female has the propensity for and is observed curving her legs open and embracing a man's thighs and buttocks, this means she has abundant qi of the tendons.

"When the female has the propensity for and is observed caressing and fondling a man's Jade Stem, this means the qi of her blood is fully enriched.

"When the female has the propensity for and is observed becoming delirious when caressing a man's chest, this means the qi of her muscles is fully replenished.

"When a female has the propensity for and is observed playing gently with her own nipples and Jade Gate, this means she seeks union with the Mysterious Ancestor [Illumination].

"If a man wishes to successfully seduce a woman, he must be fully aware and capable of applying these two aspects: he must know how and when to caress a female's neck, breasts, and vagina; and he must know how to recognize the Nine Energies of the female.

"Knowing these aspects are extremely important to ensuring a joyous sexual union with a female. However, if a female does not exhibit any of the Nine Energies, the man should apply the Nine Techniques in order to initiate a more positive effect."

The Five Signs of Female Sensuality

The Yellow Emperor asked Plain Girl, "What are the signs of a woman who is sexually aroused?"

Plain Girl responded, "When a woman begins to feel sensual, there are Five Signs that indicate her desire. Once engaged in sexual activity, the Five Desires are exhibited in her. But, Your Majesty, you must also keep in mind the Ten Movements. From the Five Signs, a man can become aware of what kind of sexual pleasure a woman wishes to share with him. Furthermore, he will be able to determine what degree of intensity is important to her for touching and what type of sexual activity she desires. The Five Signs that reveal her sexual arousal are:

"When her face and cheeks are flushed, she wishes to feel the Jade Stem in her hands and to feel it rubbing gently near her Jade

Gate. If redness appears on her upper chest, she desires to feel the Jade Stem upon her tongue.

"When her nipples harden and the nasal passages becomes moist, she wishes to feel the Jade Stem inserted gently inside her Jade Gate and wishes for intense stimulation of her clitoris.

"When her lips and throat exhibit dryness and she begins creating saliva to counter the dryness, she desires the movement of a Jade Stem inside her Jade Gate. This is also a sign that she wishes to be touched, caressed, and kissed on the neck, breasts, and Jade Gate.

"When her Jade Gate becomes moist, she desires the Jade Stem's deep and methodical penetration within her Jade Gate. Along with this she desires to be kissed passionately and to be touched sensually.

"When the secretions begin to completely flood her Jade Gate, resulting in fluids dripping down her thighs and legs, she desires the utmost intensity for the Mysterious Ancestor. The man should then slowly withdraw his Jade Stem from her Jade Gate and place it upon her Red Lotus so she can immerse herself in the sublime Tao."

The Five Desires

Plain Girl continued, "Concerning the Five Desires, these are signs exhibited in the woman once in the throes of passion and sexual activity. But each sign varies in degree depending on the intensity experienced by each individual female. Through close observation of her, the man will be able to discern the level of sensuality and sexual intensity she is experiencing, so that when she reaches the state of extreme intensity he will cease his sexual activity and leave her alone to roam freely within the sublime Tao. The Five Desires of a woman are:

"When a woman desires to be lovingly embraced, caressed, or touched, or when she desires to feel the Jade Stem, she tends to await this with bated breath and with either a rubbing or scratching movement with the hand on her upper chest and neck.

"When a woman's breasts and Jade Gate are lovingly caressed her nostrils will widen, her lips will open, her tongue will sway over the lips, and her hands will reach out to feel the Jade Stem.

"When her sexual desire becomes intense and secretions are flowing from the Jade Gate, she will want to closely embrace the man, pulling him close and tightly to her by pushing on either his back or his buttocks.

"When she reaches orgasm without engaging in intercourse, she drips with perspiration all over her body and her clothing becomes drenched.

"In the event that she achieves a heightened state of sexual stimulation and enters into a trancelike state, her body will feel extremely light, as if drifting and floating on air. Her spirit will feel as though it is above and outside her body, and her body will be so relaxed that it appears to be as still as a piece of wood. Her eyes will be closed but she will gaze upward under her lids, as she is immersed in heightened sensual bliss."

Recognizing Female Sexual Desire

The Yellow Emperor asked of Plain Girl, "You have said that along with knowing the Five Signs and Five Desires of a female I must also be aware of the Ten Movements so that the Tao can be followed. Could you please explain these Ten Movements to me?"

Plain Girl told him, "The Ten Movements that reveal a female's yin and yang aspects for desiring sexual contact are:

"When she desires to embrace the man she draws him close and presses her breasts against him and her pelvis pushes up against him rhythmically. She pants and her voice sounds uncontrollably cracked and shaky. Her tongue extends out and she seeks to lick and taste him in order to fully stimulate and excite him. These, Your Majesty, are the movements of her great arousal.

"When she lays her fragrant body back and her eyes close, her nostrils widen, she is unable to speak, she finds difficulty breathing, and her thighs and legs are held straight out, this means she desires to feel the Jade Stem stimulating her clitoris.

"When the man is sleeping and she lays her head on his thigh or stomach to sensuously stare at his Jade Stem, and then she begins to play with it by gently twisting and stroking it, this shows she is hungry for the taste and feel of his Jade Stem.

"When her face flushes, her ears redden, the tip of her tongue feels slightly colder, she moves her buttocks back and forth, her eyebrows and eyelids flicker, she voices playful words and makes groaning sounds, this shows she wishes to be submissively passionate.

"When her hands and abdomen become extremely warm and

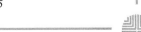

when she speaks unintelligibly and uses her hands to open her thighs, nervously opening and closing them, and she makes motions with her legs to draw the man closer, this shows that she wishes to have the Jade Stem thrust deeply into her Jade Gate.

"When her tongue extends out, her face looks as though entranced, her body is limp and relaxed, and her limbs appear to droop, this is a sign that she wishes to be sexually taken and to feel vigorous deep and shallow thrusts into her Jade Gate.

"When she leans her body nervously from side to side, stretching her toes and feet out, and she sucks the saliva within her mouth, murmurs in low tones, and makes gestures of wishing to be closer to him, this shows that the tide of yin is approaching and you should direct her to kneel between your legs so she may completely absorb your energy.

"When her vagina pulses noticeably, her secretions flood down to her inner thighs, she turns her waist from side to side, she perspires, she smiles, and her back arches, this shows she is reaching the peak of union with the yin and yang. She will not want the man to ejaculate because her desire is to prolong this sensation for as long as possible.

"When she exhibits sensuous behavior, says that she feels pleasure mounting in her, moves her body in a tossing manner, stretches out her back, and pulls at the man's skin or hair, this shows she desperately seeks to reach the peak of yin, but is not yet there.

"When her body feels hot and is dampened by perspiration, the hands and feet fall limp, and her secretions profusely flow down the inner thighs, this shows she is completely satisfied with her sensations of heightened pleasure.

"From these signs, Your Majesty, a man can clearly determine the degrees and types of sexual stimulation a woman desires."

BOOK V
Sexual Postures, Techniques, and Therapies

The Nine Sexual Positions

The Yellow Emperor said to Plain Girl, "You have given me the specific knowledge for the correct approach and behaviors for sexual activity, which also entails using nine specific positions. Please enlighten me clearly on these, so that these treasures for practicing sexual activity may be recorded for my future reference, and so I can correctly practice these precious secrets of sexual joy."

Plain Girl then detailed each sexual position for him:

"The first position is called **Soaring Dragon**. With the female lying on her back with her legs raised up and back toward her head and the feet together, the man hovers over her from behind in a crouching fashion on his knees and begins rubbing his Jade Stem over her clitoral area. When the Jade Stem is fully erect he inserts it into her Jade Gate using the Eight Shallow and Two Deep method. When the erection reaches its peak and the feeling of the pending ejaculation is experienced, he withdraws his

Jade Stem from her. When the sensation of ejaculation has sub-
sided and the erection has softened slightly, he reinserts the Jade
Stem and begins the Eight Shallow and Two Deep method again.
He repeats this procedure ten times.

"This technique will strengthen the Jade Stem and provide him
with greater staying power, and the female will experience intense
sexual pleasure from the contractions of her Jade Gate. This technique will also cure any stomach disorders either partner may be
suffering from.

"The second position is called **Forest Tigers**. The female lies
prostrate with a pillow under her stomach to raise her buttocks.
The man then positions himself on his knees behind her and
holds her by the waist with both hands. He inserts the full length
of his Jade Stem into her Jade Gate and proceeds to swiftly withdraw the entire length; he repeats this movement of the Jade Stem
thirty-six times. The man must prevent his ejaculation. After each
set of thirty-six repetitions he rests until the Jade Stem softens
slightly and there is no sensation of ejaculation, at which point he
begins the technique again. He does this ten times in succession.

"This technique will strengthen and eliminate any disorders
the man might have of the heart and liver.

"The third position is called **Playful Monkeys**. The female lies
supine with a pillow underneath her in order to slightly raise her
buttocks. She positions her thighs against her abdomen with the
calves and feet raised straight up. The man, facing her, squats over
her on his knees, with his Jade Stem positioned behind her

buttocks. Using both hands he supports her legs on his shoulders so that her knees are positioned higher than her breasts.

"The man then inserts the head of his Jade Stem into her Jade Gate and makes eight shallow thrusts. He withdraws the Jade Stem and slides the entire shaft twice along her labia and over the clitoris, as though making two deep thrusts. He then inserts the head of the Jade Stem, repeating this procedure ten times.

"After the ten repetitions are complete, he inserts the Jade Stem even deeper into her (about three inches) and repeats the same procedure another ten times. Finally, he inserts the full length of his Jade Stem and repeats the procedure ten times or until the woman reaches orgasm.

"This method will increase the hardness of erections, lengthen staying power, strengthen the spirit, and benefit longevity.

"The fourth position is called **Mating Cicadas**. The woman lies face down, with the legs held straight and together. The man squats over her and gently leans on her back while inserting his Jade Stem into her Jade Gate. She should attempt to raise her buttocks slightly so as to better feel the sensations of penetration upon the labia. He thrusts his Jade Stem into her fifty-four times.

"During the man's thrusting, she alternates vaginal contractions with his thrusts and dilation during his retreats. After fifty-four repetitions he rests momentarily, and then begins again. When the woman reaches orgasm the procedure ends.

"This technique will rid both of them of the seven emotional illnesses: depression, anger, sorrow, selfishness, remorse, fear, and nervousness.

"The fifth position is called **Floating Tortoises**. The woman lies on her back with her buttocks rolled up off the bed and her knees positioned up and over her breasts. The man kneels over her, drawing his body close to hers, and inserts his Jade Stem into her Jade Gate. With both hands he gently holds her legs back. With his Jade Stem he stimulates both the Jade Gate and her clitoris, inserting the Jade Stem, withdrawing it and letting it slide over her clitoral area, and inserting it again. He does this repeatedly until her secretions are flowing.

"When the woman begins grinding her pelvis from the intense stimulation of her Jade Gate, the man should then deeply thrust his Jade Stem into her and continue thrusting until she orgasms. He then stops.

"This technique will make the man physically stronger and increase his vitality. It is also used for dispelling unwanted toxins in the five organs.

"The sixth position is called **Flying Phoenixes**. The woman lies on her back with her legs held apart and bent at the knees. The man kneels between her legs and supports his body by placing his forearms on the bed on either side of her. His inserts his Jade Stem deeply into her Jade Gate once, then withdraws it to slide back and forth across her vaginal area nine times. During the deep insertion of the Jade Stem the woman should make short, rhythmic rocking movements to press the Jade Stem deep within her; she does this twenty-four times. This will cause her secretions to gush.

"The woman must be sure that she contracts her thighs around the man's waist when he has thrust his Jade Stem deeply within her, and relaxes the thighs when he has withdrawn and is stimulating the outside of her Jade Gate.

"When she reaches orgasm the man will cease having intercourse with her. With frequent use of this method the qi in the marrow of the bones will be benefited.

"The seventh position is called **Licking Rabbits**. The man lies upon his back with his legs together and straight out. The woman mounts him, facing away from him, her knees bent and the legs held along the man's sides and under his shoulders. She places most of her weight on her knees and legs, supporting herself with her hands and arms, and allows her head to droop downward.

"The man's Jade Stem is inserted deeply into her Jade Gate. She uses any motions of her choosing to stimulate herself and to cause her secretions to gush forth. When she orgasms, the intercourse is stopped. This technique will avoid the onset of any illness in the man.

"The eighth position is called **Diving Fish**. The man lies on his back with his legs together and straight out. The woman mounts him, sitting atop his forelegs and facing him. Bending her knees with her legs extended out alongside his, she rests her weight on her knees and legs.

"She then moves her buttocks forward, gradually allowing the head of his Jade Stem to enter her Jade Gate. However, deep penetration is not allowed, and she must control the depth throughout. She uses any motion of her choosing to maintain shallow penetration, much like a baby suckling upon a nipple but not engulfing the entire breast.

"During this technique the man is to remain motionless and allow the woman to make the movements, which helps make the act of intercourse last longer. When she reaches orgasm, the Jade Stem is withdrawn. This exercise will prevent many types of ailments in the man.

"The ninth position is called **Crane Necking**. While facing the woman, the man kneels with his knees held open and thighs spread apart. The female kneels in front of him with her thighs positioned on either side of his and her hands and arms placed around and behind his head.

"The man's Jade Stem is inserted into her Jade Gate, and the shaft will rub her labia and stimulate her clitoris. The man places both his hands on her buttocks to guide the up and down movements and to ensure deep penetration.

"When the woman orgasms, the intercourse is stopped. With this technique all the Seven Traumas shall be eradicated in the man."

The Eight Benefits

Plain Girl told the Yellow Emperor, "Sexual activity between a man and a woman can have both positive benefits and negative effects. If sexual activity is practiced in accordance with balancing the qi, diseases of the body and mind can be prevented and health can be maintained at its optimum. I will now explain the benefits and techniques.

"The first technique is called **Strengthening the Ching**. The woman lies on her right side with her legs stretched out and slightly bent at the knees. The man lies on his left side in the same manner but with his head near her legs. They are lying opposite each other and facing one another's genitals. The man places his middle finger inside the woman's Jade Gate and makes eighteen deep and rhythmic thrusts into her. The woman places his Jade Stem in her mouth, and in unison with the man's thrusts she makes eighteen in-and-out deep sucking motions.

"Doing this exercise two times per day for fifteen consecutive days will eliminate and prevent any abnormalities in the circulatory system. It will also thicken the man's semen and prevent the woman from experiencing excessively heavy menstrual periods."

"The second method is called **Harmonizing the Qi.** The woman lies on her back, supporting her head high up on a cushion, and spreads her legs wide. The man then kneels between her legs and supports himself with his hands and arms.

"Just the head of the Jade Stem is placed inside the Jade Gate, and the man then makes twenty-seven slow and gentle thrusts. After this, intercourse ceases.

"To ensure the efficacy of this method, it should be performed three times a day for twenty-one consecutive days. This technique rids the mind of all tension and regulates the pulses. It can also help cure frigidity in women.

"The third technique is called **Accumulating Ching.** The woman lies on her right side with the knees slightly bent and with her body in a v-shape. The man lies on his right side directly behind her, placing his left hand on her left hip and waist.

"The man then slides his Jade Stem through her closed legs and makes thirty-six thrusts against her labia. The woman simultaneously stimulates the head of his Jade Stem with her left fingers. If Dragon Rain appears at the tip of his Jade Stem, she should retrieve it with her left index finger and place it on her tongue for ingestion.

"Practice this method four times a day for twenty consecutive days. This technique will strengthen a man's sexual energy so that it can be increased and developed in his body, thus creating a calm mind and relaxed body. In women it cures and prevents frigidity. Keep in mind that ejaculation is not to occur.

"The fourth method is called **Bone Strengthening**. The woman lies on her right side, bringing her left knee up toward her chest and supporting it with both arms. She then extends the left leg and foot out. The man hovers over her from behind, supporting himself on his knees and arms. He then inserts the head of his Jade Stem into her Jade Gate and performs forty-five slow rhythmic thrusts. When the thrusts are finished, the intercourse is over.

"Practice this five times daily for ten consecutive days. This technique aids in strengthening the marrow of the bones and will help lubricate and keep pliable all the joints of the body. It will also encourage relaxation and mental stability and will help remove diseases in the body, especially chronic amenorrhea in women.

"The fifth technique is called **Harmonizing the Pulses**. The woman lies on her right side, bringing her right knee up toward her chest and supporting it with both arms. She extends the right leg and foot out. The man hovers over her from behind, supporting himself on his hands and knees. He then inserts the head of his Jade Stem into her Jade Gate and performs fifty-four slow rhythmic thrusts. When the thrusting is finished intercourse is over.

"Practice this six times daily for twenty consecutive days. This technique will regulate the man's pulses so they remain even and regular. In women the method will cure or prevent hyperkinesis.

"The sixth method is called **Purifying the Blood.** The woman and man kneel in front of each other, with the woman's legs opened and positioned outside the man's legs, which are held together. The man holds her waist and hips with both hands, and she rests her hands upon his shoulders. His Jade Stem is inserted deeply into her Jade Gate. She makes thirty-six sensuous grinding motions with her hips and pelvis.

"The man then lies back and the woman bends over to place the head of his Jade Stem into her mouth, performing thirty-six complete circlings around the head of his Jade Stem with her tongue. She simultaneously applies a tight and constant sucking action with her mouth.

"The woman then lies back with her knees held up near her breasts with her hands and arms, her legs and thighs held open. With the fingers of both hands the man opens her labia so that he can engulf her entire vaginal area with his mouth. He then performs forty-eight in-and-out sucking motions with his mouth.

"To ensure the efficacy of this technique it must be performed seven times a day for ten days. This technique will greatly aid in stimulating the man's circulation, increasing the size of his glans penis, and strengthening his constitution. For the woman, this technique helps her vagina to be more sensitive, increases her blood circulation, and prevents irregular menstruation.

"The seventh method is called **Nourishing the Ching**. The woman crouches down on her stomach with a large cushion placed under her so that her buttocks are raised high and her labia protrudes, allowing easy access for the man's Jade Stem. The man positions himself behind her, supporting himself on his hands and knees. He then proceeds to use the Nine Shallow and One Deep method in eight consecutive rounds.

"To ensure efficacy of this method it must be performed eight times a day for ten consecutive days. This technique will strengthen the entire skeletal structure of both the man and the woman, and it will enrich their endocrine systems.

"The eighth technique is called **Refining the Three Treasures**. The woman lies on her back and draws up her legs with the knees bent and legs held together. The heels of her feet should be brought up to touch her buttocks. The palms of both her hands are placed firmly over her ears. The man kneels facing her and crouches over her with her knees pressing against his chest and his hands positioned on either side of her to support his weight. He then inserts the head of his Jade Stem into her Jade Gate and makes use of the Nine Shallow and One Deep technique nine consecutive times. Then the intercourse is stopped.

"This technique should be performed nine times a day for ten consecutive days. It will balance and enrich the ching, qi, and shen of both partners, as well as cure any offensive vaginal odor in the female."

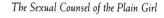

The Seven Traumas

Plain Girl then went on to explain to the Yellow Emperor, "If sexual activity is not performed with the principles of properly balancing the qi, it will create traumas in both the body and mind. Therefore, I will give you a detailed explanation of the Seven Traumas and their cures.

"The first trauma is called **Extinguishing Ching**. It is called this because it is associated with the vital energy being dried up and resembles the smothering of a candle flame. It occurs when the sex drive becomes insufficient in strength yet sexual activity is still engaged in. When attempting sex this trauma will cause the body to sweat profusely and will create a feeling of lost energy and stamina—despite feeling mentally excited. It will cause you to close your eyes while trying desperately to bring about a strong enough erection so sex can be performed.

"To cure this trauma, the woman lies on her back and the man positions himself behind and over her head so that his Jade Stem can be taken into her mouth. With her left hand she lightly grips and pulls down on his scrotum. With the head of the Jade Stem in her mouth, she makes small circles with her head as she rhythmically encircles the head of the Jade Stem with her tongue. She does this until the Jade Stem is erect but does not allow ejaculation to occur.

"Do this nine times per day for ten days.

"The second trauma is called **Overflowing Ching**. It is called this because it refers to a man with a high sex drive who has not harmonized the aspects of yin and yang within his sexual activity, and who therefore experiences premature ejaculation—and in many cases ejaculates before having reached full erection.

"In connection with this problem, if sexual activity is engaged in while the man is drunk it will produce a shortness of breath, which can damage his lungs. Other ill effects include erratic coughing, pinkeye, a frequent dry throat, urinary problems, depression, anxiety, and an explosive temper. Over an extended period of time the dryness of the throat will be followed by a fever, after which the man will suffer from impotence.

"To cure and prevent this trauma, the woman lies on her back and embraces the man's waist with her legs. He positions himself over her and between her legs, supporting his weight with his knees and hands. He then inserts his Jade Stem into her Jade Gate at a maximum depth of two inches. During intercourse she matches his movements by raising her buttocks when he thrusts inward and lowering her buttocks when he moves up and out. These movements are continued in unison until the woman begins salivating profusely. At this point intercourse is stopped.

"To achieve the optimum therapeutic effect, the man must prevent ejaculation. Perform this technique nine times per day for ten consecutive days.

"The third trauma is called **Disrupted Pulse**. It is called this because it is associated with having an irregular pulse rate, which feels disrupted or erratic. This can be caused by having sex when the Jade Stem has not reached full erection. This indiscriminate use of the Jade Stem will cause premature ejaculation midway through sexual activity, and so causes a loss of stamina in the male. The problem can also result from engaging in sexual activity when the stomach is still full, which causes damage to the spleen. If the man likewise suffers from indigestion the Jade Stem will shrink and his virility will diminish.

"To cure and prevent this trauma, the woman lies on her back and embraces the man's waist with her legs. He positions himself over her and between her legs, supporting his weight with his knees and hands. He then inserts his Jade Stem into her Jade Gate and makes use of the Nine Shallow and One Deep technique until she reaches orgasm. Intercourse is then stopped.

"To achieve the optimum therapeutic effect of this method the man must prevent ejaculation. Perform this technique nine times per day for ten consecutive days.

"The fourth trauma is called **Vanishing Ching**. It is called this because it is associated with feeling as if the sexual energy has leaked away. It is a result of mental and physical exhaustion and fatigue, which causes poor production of semen. When a man is tired and lacks stamina yet hurriedly attempts sexual activity without allowing time for his sweat to dry and to restore his energy, he will experience a feverish feeling in his stomach and his lips will become extremely dry.

"To cure and prevent this trauma, the man lies on his back and stretches out his legs. The woman positions herself over him, straddling his legs and facing him while supporting her weight on her knees, shins, and hands. With the Jade Stem inserted in her Jade Gate, she then makes up-and-down movements with her buttocks while he lies still. Once she reaches orgasm, intercourse is stopped.

"To achieve the optimum therapeutic effect of this method the man must prevent ejaculation. Perform this technique nine times per day for ten consecutive days.

"The fifth trauma is called **Dysfunctioning Organs.** It is called this because it is associated with ailments of the heart, spleen, lungs, kidneys, and liver. A man who has ailments of the internal organs will more often than not have difficulties associated with defecation and urination. If engaging in sexual activity before restoring himself, he will cause injury to his liver. Even if he limits the time he spends engaged in sexual activity, he will further his suffering by causing muscular fatigue, blurred vision, and decreased the blood circulation. If he continues to engage in sexual activity he will experience acute muscle spasms, impotence, and the inability to achieve erection.

"To cure and prevent this trauma, the man lies on his back and stretches out his legs. The woman positions herself over him, straddling his legs and facing him while supporting her weight with her knees, shins, and hands. She leans slightly forward toward his face, allowing the Jade Stem to enter her Jade Gate at a depth of only two inches, and then makes gentle gyrating movements with her buttocks while he lies still. Once she reaches orgasm, intercourse is stopped.

"To achieve the optimum therapeutic effect of this method the man must prevent ejaculation. Perform this technique nine times per day for ten consecutive days.

"The sixth trauma is called **One Hundred Obstructions**. This means that all the pulses of the body are blocked. The primary cause of this trauma is a man choosing a female partner who lacks sexual restraint, is extremely lustful, and craves multiple sexual encounters that end with his ejaculation. Because of this he becomes completely bereft of ching, and despite his eagerness to please his partner he loses his ability to ejaculate. He will soon suffer the complications of extreme dryness of the throat, inability to urinate, and frequent dizziness accompanied by headaches.

"To cure and prevent this trauma, the man lies on his back and stretches out his legs. The woman positions herself over him, straddling his legs and facing away from him while supporting her weight with her knees, shins, and hands. She leans forward slightly, allowing the Jade Stem to enter her Jade Gate at full depth, and then makes gentle gyrating movements with her buttocks while he lies still. Once she reaches orgasm, intercourse is stopped.

"To achieve the optimum therapeutic effect of this method the man must prevent ejaculation. Perform this technique nine times per day for ten consecutive days.

"The seventh trauma is called **Weakened Blood**. When the man is exhausted and perspiring from the day's work yet still engages in sexual activity, his blood will become weakened. Even though one encounter under these conditions may not be that damaging, multiple encounters that end with his ejaculating will diminish his ching and over time will cause him to suffer other ailments such as painful urination, anemia, painful nocturnal emissions and paling of the complexion. The Jade Stem will take on a wet and sticky feel because the urine will show traces of blood mixing with semen.

"To cure and prevent this trauma, the woman lies on her back, with a cushion under her buttocks to raise them and her legs spread as widely as possible to accommodate the man. As he kneels between her legs he holds the backs of her knee joints with both hands and raises them up to accommodate his thrusting. He then inserts his Jade Stem into her Jade Gate and makes use of the Nine Shallow and One Deep technique until she reaches orgasm. Intercourse is then stopped.

"To achieve the optimum therapeutic effect of this method the man must prevent ejaculation. Perform this technique nine times per day for ten consecutive days."

Efficacious Method for Impregnating

Plain Girl then told the Yellow Emperor, "There are established guidelines for ensuring the impregnation of a woman. The most important and initial condition is that she must be physically healthy and emotionally tranquil, without any feelings of depression or stress. Make sure she is neatly dressed in bedchamber garments and has adhered to a vegetarian diet for the preceding twenty-four days.

"Three days after the completion of her menstrual period between the hours of midnight and the cock crowing at dawn, the woman should be engaged in sexual intercourse.

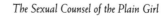

"Most importantly, be patient. Allow adequate time in which to stimulate her and follow the principles of yin-yang love techniques. Doing so will ensure that both partners experience the joys and pleasures of an intense encounter. At the time when the man is to ejaculate, it is extremely important that he does not withdraw the Jade Stem too quickly. If the Jade Stem is withdrawn too quickly it will sever the energies and the connection of the Jade Stem to the uterus, and this will cause the sperm to not enter the woman's uterus properly.

"Should the woman become pregnant from making use of this method, the child will be exceptional and well-gifted and assured of a long life."

The Six Sexual Taboos for Men

Plain Girl again spoke: "The proper application of yin-yang techniques requires that both the man and woman observe certain taboos. If a man is at his peak energy and vitality and impregnates a woman, that child will, more often than not, inherit good health and a long life. If an elderly man whose sexual energy is not vital impregnates a woman, that child will, more often than not, be of ill health and have a short life. So the most important concern is the sexual energy of the man.

"There are many men who are sexually overindulgent and they die an untimely death. Therefore, in order to live a long and healthy life men should not be sexually overindulgent. It is this fact that is of the greatest importance to men.

"If a man does become ill from overindulgence he must take

the proper herbal medicines to affect a cure. However, he should play close attention to refraining from violating the following six taboos. If he does adhere to not violating the taboos, he will eliminate all the ill effects and his sexual vitality will be restored."

The First Taboo

"On the last day of the full moon and the first day of the crescent moon, sexual activity should be avoided. Sexual acts performed on these days will produce children with damaged vital energy (qi). Also, if a man violates this taboo, when he later desires sexual activity he will suffer from the inability to produce a full erection. Even though he may burn with desire, the result will be a reddish-yellow color to the urine and nocturnal emissions of watery semen. Hence his life span will be shortened."

The Second Taboo

"No sexual activity is to be performed during storms of rain, lightning, or thunder or during any severe inclement weather and earthquakes. Children conceived during these circumstances can be born insane, deaf, dumb, or blind or be born mentally ill or full of grief and constant worry. If the man engages in sexual activity during these circumstances he cannot enter into any spiritual realms, and this will adversely affect his qi and shen."

The Third Taboo

"No sexual activity is to be performed on a full stomach or when the man has drunk excessively; the internal organs can be damaged,

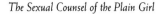

resulting in reddish urination, pallor, lower back pain, lumbago, edema, and severe indigestion—all of which will shorten a man's life."

The Fourth Taboo

"There should be no sexual activity until thirty minutes after urination when the body is restored to normalcy. Otherwise this could result in severe indigestion, loss of appetite, swelling in the abdominal region, and melancholia—which will cause emotional irritability and unstableness, to the point of appearing in his actions to be insane."

The Fifth Taboo

"There should be no sexual activity while a man is recuperating from fatigue or an illness; he must fully restore his strength first. If this taboo is not followed he will tend to have shortness of breath, constant thirst, indigestion, and pain throughout his muscles and joints."

The Sixth Taboo

"On the occasion when the man is exposed to a woman who engages in obscene and rude conversation, if he experiences an erection during their conversation he is to avoid having sexual activity. If he violates this taboo the Jade Stem will suffer from aches, his internal organs will suffer from traumas, his eyes and ears will suffer various problems, he will develop a severe cough, his mind will suffer from lack of clarity, and he may even experience impotence.

"Hence, the man who continually violates these taboos is but destined to be an invalid, becoming infirm and totally dependent on spirit-blessed herbal medicines."

FIVE

Reverting Ching to the Brain

(The Yellow Stream or Stream of Life)

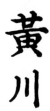

No one saw me paddling upon the Yellow Stream
or slicing the bright moon upon a shimmering mirror.
But when the wind was heard, I sang
and herons flew over rejoicing in kind.
The affect of the Yellow Stream felt so joyous and contented,
it was as if I was drunk and slept happily embracing a crane of
immortality.
Ask all those who just seek gold and fame,
Have they not read Chuang Chou's "Autumn Waters"?

—White Tigress Manual

In Taoist practices there are two primary stages males must go through in order to create the Elixir of Immortality. The first stage is Opening the Original Cavity, and it is accomplished through meditation or contemplation. For White Tigresses, Opening the

Original Cavity occurs more readily during her practice of Absorbing Male Sexual Energy. The second stage men must complete is stimulating the Yellow Stream (also called Reverting Ching to the Brain, or in some Taoist sects, the Stream of Life). White Tigresses refer to this experience as Illumination and One Hundred Returnings.

Later in the alchemical process men need to have successful mobilization of qi through the River Cart, which in Taoist books is also called the Lesser Heavenly Circuit. From this experience the Taoist male is able to begin the work of completing nine such circuits of qi, called the Nine Returnings, so that he may refine and deposit one drop of pure elixir into his abdomen (*tan t'ien*) and form the spiritual embryo. At this point his immortal spirit is formed and will begin to be developed and strengthened, not unlike the pregnancy of the female, thus transforming the male into an immortal.

The section that follows details the Yellow Stream, as this is the central experience to which White Tigresses and Jade Dragons aspire. It will be assumed that serious male Taoist practitioners are already working toward the state of Opening the Original Cavity in their meditation practice, as described in chapter 5.

The following is a translation of a section in the *White Tigress Manual*, but these teachings originally appeared in the biography of the Han dynasty Taoist adept P'ei Hsuan-jen, which was written by Teng Yun-tzu of the Tang dynasty. The original is filled with many cryptic Taoist terms so I am translating this text in a freer manner so the reader can better understand it. This text is important to all Taoists who practice sexual and alchemical methods, and it is especially important to any man who undertakes the role of a Jade Dragon with a White Tigress; it is paramount to his progress with

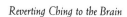

the Transformational Techniques that are described in *The Sexual Teachings of the White Tigress*.

Discourse on the Yellow Stream
(Reverting Ching to the Brain)

After having concentrated and purified their thoughts [through meditation], the man and woman may begin practicing the art that will lead them to longevity. But this method should only be transmitted to adepts and kept secret from all others. It will allow a man and woman together to stimulate and mobilize their qi, so the man may nurture his ching [semen and sexual energy] and the woman her blood [the origin of her sexual energy]. This is not a heterodox method, as it focuses on activating the yin [in males] and strengthening the yang [in females]. If this discipline is practiced in the correct manner the qi fluid [blood] will freely circulate like clouds throughout the entire body and the seed [the essence of the elixir] will congeal and become harmonious. Briefly, all those who practice this, whether young or old, will begin to feel like adolescents.

The two partners should first begin by meditating, detaching their minds from their bodies and worldly matters. They should then grind their teeth together seven times [and then engage in sexual activity for stimulation of the ching and qi].

[Having had sexual stimulation and the moments preceding

each of their orgasms], the man applies pressure to his penis and locks his semen from escaping, so that the accumulated qi can ascend along the spinal column until it reaches the *ni-wan* cavity at the top of the brain. This is called Returning to the Origin.

The woman controls her passionate emotions and nurtures her spirit so that she does not physically gyrate in her climax, so the refined fire does not move. She causes the qi of her two breasts to descend [into the kidney area] and then causes it to ascend into her *ni-wan* cavity. This is called Transforming the True.

The elixir will thus be formed [in both participants] if nurtured for one hundred days, and so each will fully retain his or her spiritual vitality. If continued over a very long period the experience [of the Yellow Stream] will happen naturally, as will longevity and attaining immortality.

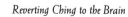

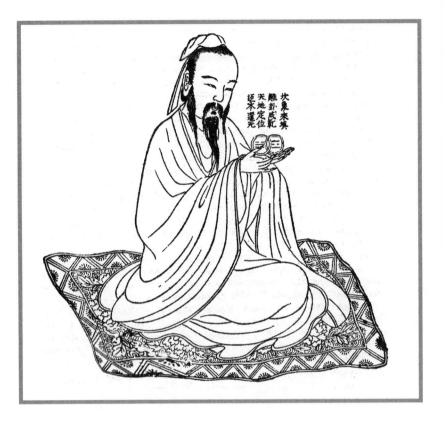

Balancing Yin and Yang

A Taoist adept shown balancing the male (Li/Fire image in his left hand) and female (K'an/Water image in his right hand) principles. From the Ming dynasty.

The Chinese verse reads:

> *Within the image of Water comes forth fulfillment.*
> *Within the image of Fire creation is completed.*
> *Heaven and Earth are then in their proper positions,*
> *Returning to the Source is then assured.*

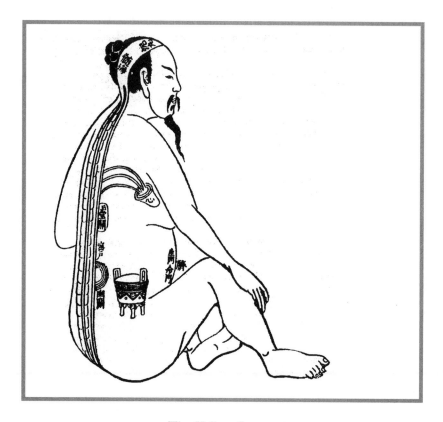

The Yellow Stream

(*Huang Chuan*)

A Ming dynasty diagram showing the path of the Yellow Stream up a Taoist adept's spine. The Chinese characters in the diagram indicate the following (starting with the topmost upon the head): *ni-wan* (literally "mud ball") and below *sui hai* (the brain, but literally translates as "ocean of marrow"). It is the *ni-wan* that creates the illumination when the ching is reverted up into the brain. In the middle of the spine the characters indicate an area called *hu tang kuan* (Door of the Hall Passage) and below that is the *chueh hu* (Secret Door) and the *yu kuan* (Secret Passage). In front of the abdomen are the characters *sheng men* (Gate of Birth) and *ming men* (Gate of Life).

Commentary

The preceding text needs clarification, as those not steeped in Taoist ideology will be somewhat lost. Even though there is a technique involved, the main way of and catalyst for experiencing illumination is actually sexual intensity. Each partner must seek to fully stimulate the other and themselves so that the necessary sexual excitement is produced. These are not just rote techniques; they only produce an effect if the intensity reaches the highest level possible.

The first, and most important, idea is that a man conserves and retains his semen and sexual energy, literally preventing his ejaculation at the very moment preceding orgasm. He obstructs the semen from being ejaculated by tightly pressing his left index finger and thumb to the base of his penis while his right hand pinches the tip of his glans penis. He also holds his breath until the sensation of climax ends, simultaneously closing in his anal muscles to block any escape of the energy. At the same time he rolls his eyes upward as if to view his brain. He then maintains an extended exhalation as he mentally draws his semen back into the kidney area and then up along the spinal column until it reaches the brain, or *ni-wan* cavity, and creates the Illumination effect.

Obviously it is not the semen that is actually drawn up into the brain, but rather the energy of his pending orgasm. This technique is very difficult to master, and each man must find his own best body position and sexual act in order to properly practice this. It must be made clear, however, that the technique is useless unless it is undertaken by a man and woman of compatible natures. This is also not a rote sexual technique, and it depends greatly on the trust and emotions between the two partners; without the ability to be totally relaxed and comfortable with each other, the tension of unfamiliarity will prevent the qi from being stimulated properly. The whole technique is based on borrowing and harmonizing the essence of the other person, yin and yang replenishing each other. The texts also warn against performing this technique while intoxicated. It should also never be attempted with masturbation alone, as this will harm the body's essences and result in no benefit.

The woman controls her emotions at the very moment preceding her orgasm. She does allow her orgasm to occur, but restrains the physical effects of it as best she can by calming her mind and focusing on the qi in her breasts. At the moment preceding orgasm she places her index fingers and thumbs over the bottom portion of each respective nipple and areola, applying pressure with her fingertips. She simultaneously crosses or squeezes her legs together tightly so her essence does not escape—which is what is meant by "the refined fire does not move." While doing this, she focuses on her qi descending from her breasts into her kidney region. With the tongue placed upon the roof of her mouth and her eyes gazing back and up to internally view her brain, she visualizes the qi rising up her spinal column into her *ni-wan* cavity. As with men, she must also find the best body position and sexual act in which to practice this technique.

The next step is in the nurturing process. "For one hundred days following the experience of the Yellow Stream" means that during each day of that period both partners will attempt to recreate the effect again. Whether or not it happens is irrelevant, as the emphasis is on nurturing the ching and qi. This also means that periodically each partner may fully experience orgasm, but if the orgasm is to be released each must wait until the third sensation of orgasm before releasing his or her sexual secretions and fluids.

When sexual encounters are not possible the alternative method is to sit in meditation and mentally recreate the effect as best as possible. Those who continue to practice this way over a long period of time are said to create in themselves the Elixir of Longevity and Immortality because the ching and qi become more and more refined and will actually move the qi through the Lesser Heavenly Circuit. Hence, once the Lesser Heavenly Circuit can be performed then the work of the Nine Returnings is undertaken.

With nine successive circulations of qi through the meridians

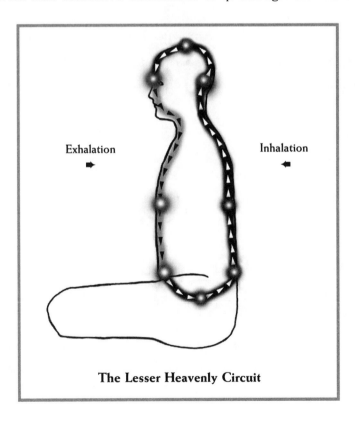

The Lesser Heavenly Circuit

tumo and *jenmo*, a drop of pure elixir (the refined ching, qi, and shen) will attach itself to the *tan t'ien*, thus creating the spiritual embryo and nurturing the spiritual fetus.

Sexual Positions for Inducing the Yellow Stream

The following are three sexual positions that the *White Tigress Manual* recommends as the most conducive for males' experiencing the Yellow Stream. In each case the actual physical movements should be gentle, slow, and rhythmic so the partners can enter a state of tranquillity and ease during the sexual stimulation. Hard or physically demanding movements will only obstruct the occurrence of Illumination, and so should be avoided throughout the encounter.

Each posture has its own sexual movements and procedures, which are best adhered to for increasing the chances of experiencing Illumination. However, since each person's body type and sense of rhythm is different it is advisable for each couple to find what works best for them.

As previously stated, ideally each partner will not climax until the third sensation of orgasm is experienced, using the first two sensations as a means for inducing Illumination. If Illumination is not experienced after two sensations of pending climax, the orgasm should be released on the third occasion.

Tigress Coils the Dragon

With the man sitting upright on the edge of the bed, the female lies behind his back and wraps her body around his waist. Her right

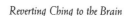

hand holds and stimulates the penis and her left fingers move gently up along his spine from the tailbone up to the Double Pass (middle of the spinal column) to aid in the upward movement of qi. There is no downward movement, only upward.

She then applies her lips, tongue, and mouth to his glans penis to stimulate and maintain his erection. Her right hand gently strokes the penis shaft.

The man, sitting upright, places his left fingers on the woman's vulva and vaginal opening, stimulating around her clitoris with small, gentle circular movements. He cups his right palm over her ear so that she can hear the internal sounds of her blood and qi, as if listening to a seashell.

At the moment preceding either the male or female orgasm, they revert to the techniques and principles mentioned above.

Tigress in the Forest

The man lies on his back at the edge of the bed. The female places her right leg over his left thigh, and keeping her left foot on the floor supports herself with both hands on the bed. The man then wraps and crosses his legs around her torso while simultaneously placing his right hand along the right side of her body to help maintain her movements. His left fingers move gently up along her spine from the tailbone to the Double Pass to aid in the upward movement of qi. There is no downward movement, only upward.

After the man guides his penis into the woman's vagina, she makes gentle movements up and down on his penis, performing nine shallow penetrations (at about half the length of the penis) and one deep (full insertion of the penis). The entire time they both stimulate each other's mouths, faces, and necks with their tongues and lips.

At the moment preceding either one's orgasms, they revert to the techniques and principles outlined above.

Dragon Enters the Tigress' Cave

The female sits on the edge of the bed and opens her legs for the man, who stands between them. Once he has inserted his penis into her vagina she crosses her legs and wraps them around his torso, using her right hand on the bed behind her for support. She places her left hand on the upper part of his spine, making small up-and-down movements to stimulate the rising of his qi.

The man places his hands and arms around her waist to support his movements. He makes nine shallow penetrations and one deep penetration into her vagina. The entire time they both stimulate each other's mouths, faces, and necks with their tongues and lips.

At the moment preceding either one's orgasm, they then revert to the techniques and principles outlined above.

Reverting the Energy of Erections

Upon waking and even during meditation a male can experience an erection. It is crucial that he learn how to revert the sexual energy of this in order to forward his progress. When this happens he should grind the teeth together seven times and then place the tongue on the roof of the mouth. Next he should firmly hold the base of the penis with his left hand, applying a firm squeezing to the underside of the base. With the right index finger and thumb, he firmly—but not so hard as to cause pain or bruising of the glans penis—pinches the tip of the penis. At the same time he concentrates his breath in the lower abdomen. Upon inhalation he senses the sexual energy moving into the kidney area, and upon exhalation he senses it moving up along the spine and into the topmost portion of the brain. He repeats this breathing procedure until the erection has subsided.

It is very important that the male adheres to this practice. Erections that occur during rest and sleep are the most useful and effective for reverting sexual energy back into the body. This is true because the body is just coming out of a state of complete relaxation, the mind is tranquil, and the blood flow is stable.

The Original Cavity

Gazing upon the Green Dragon reveals the yin;
gazing into the dragon's eye reveals the yang.
Uniting them, the dragon can ride the Yellow Stream
back to its origin.

—White Tigress Manual

In forming the Elixir of Immortality, the first step, especially for males, is to achieve a level of tranquillity during meditation so that the methods contained in this section and the previous chapter can be fully realized. What the male initially seeks in these practices is both realizing the flow of qi in the body and experiencing Reverting Ching to the Brain. With these two processes completed, the male practitioner is well on the way to forming the Elixir of Immortality within himself.

Let me make clear, however, that there are two paths by which to achieve the goals of Opening the Original Cavity and Reverting Ching to the Brain. The first is the practice of seated meditation, which entails the contemplation practices described in this chapter. The second is the practice of Gazing at the Green Dragon, which is the use of sexual intensity and concentration during a voyeuristic encounter in which the White Tigress is engaged in sexual activity with a Green Dragon.

Both methods are described in this volume, as some males may have a preference for one over the other. Keep in mind that both practices can be used simultaneously if the man feels they are not contradictory.

Opening the Original Cavity

The Original Cavity (*tsu ch'iao*), some-
times called the Ancestral Hall, is located in the center of the brain, between and behind the eyes. Stimulating this cavity is essential for the development of the internal spiritual energies—ching, qi, and shen (the Three Treasures)—and the Elixir of Immortality. When concentrating on the spot between the two eyes, a light, usually in the form of white flashes, will manifest. This is the first

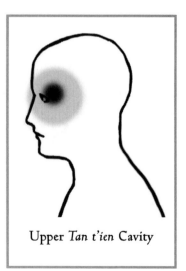

Upper *Tan t'ien* Cavity

indicator that the forming the Elixir of Immortality is beginning.

The process for Opening the Original Cavity is not complicated, but it will take patience and disciplined effort over a long
period of time. The actual method simply entails focusing all your
attention on the cavity in the center of the brain. Below are instructions for body postures, hand positions, and breathing methods for
this process.

Connected to the Original Cavity are two minor qi meridians
that branch out to the left and right sides. The left one is called *t'ai
chi* (Supreme Ultimate) and the right one is called *ch'ung ling* (Imma-
terial Spirit). They are both linked to the *t'ien ku* (Heavenly Valley)
cavity directly over them and to the *yung chuan* (Bubbling Spring)
cavities in the center of both feet. By stimulating the Original Cavity and seeing the Illumination, the qi will begin to move through
the two minor meridians, *t'ai chi* and *ch'ung ling*, and so affect the
movement of qi into the *t'ien ku* and *yung chuan* cavities. But this
movement is not something the practitioner induces; it will occur
naturally just from stimulating and opening the Original Cavity. I
mention this because when the Original Cavity begins to open you
will sense the qi moving through these two minor meridians and
then into the *t'ien ku* and *yung chuan* cavities.

The heart of this method, however, lies in two ideas, namely
that the shen (spirit or mind energy, which stimulates the Original
Cavity) resides in the mind and is exhibited in the eyes and that the
qi (vitality and breath energy, which stimulates the *tan t'ien*) resides
in the lower abdomen and expresses itself in the genitals. This is
very important to remember because without the ability to focus the
mind the Original Cavity cannot be illuminated; without keeping

the breath in the lower abdomen the genitals will lose their vigor, as the ching cannot be accumulated. The method relies heavily on the ability to concentrate on the Original Cavity and simultaneously keep the breath low in the abdomen. If this is accomplished the qi of the *t'ai chi* and *ch'ung ling* meridians will move to activate the *t'ien ku* and *yung chuan* cavities. This will benefit the practitioner with improved health, longevity, and increased sexual prowess, even in old age.

The practice of this method is purely internal and can be performed in several positions, such as sitting cross-legged, lying on the right side, lying on the back, and sitting on the edge of a chair or bed. The only real requirements are that the spine is straight and relaxed and the body is relaxed. It is also imperative that this method be practiced in a quiet and clean place, so that the mind is not distracted by external surroundings.

When comfortable and ready to begin, roll the tip of the tongue to the roof of the mouth and hold it there during the whole process. Next, lower the eyelids until just a bit of light can be seen. Direct the gaze of both eyes to the tip of the nose, focusing your mind on the spot directly between the eyes. Directing the gaze at the tip of the nose is not intended to strain the eyes, but to maintain the correct position of the eyes and eyelids in alignment with the Original Cavity.

Body Postures

If using the cross-legged seated posture, place the left leg close to and outside the right one, drawing the right heel into the perineum. The thumb and middle finger of the left hand should be joined, and the right palm should be placed underneath the left hand, bringing the thumb of the right hand up and into the middle of the left palm. Rest the hands on the lower abdomen.

If using the supine position, lie down on the right side of the body—lying on the left will put too much pressure on the heart. Cross the left ankle over the right ankle and bend the knees slightly to make the position more comfortable. The right palm should be placed under the right ear, and the left palm should be placed along the right thigh.

If lying on the back, keep the legs together and place the left hand over the lower abdomen and the right palm over the back of the left hand.

If sitting on the edge of a bed, keep the legs slightly apart and use the hand positioning explained in the cross-legged seated posture.

It is up to each individual to decide which posture best suits him. The important part is to devote at least twenty minutes twice per day to the practice. Some people actually practice all four postures each day, using one posture in the early morning, another in mid-morning, another in midafternoon, and another at bedtime.

Breathing

Breathing is the very foundation of all meditation practices. There are several disciplines applied in these practices. The first is what is called the Cleansing Breath. It requires two distinct methods and should be performed before engaging in any of the methods described in this book, whether a sexual practice or not.

The first part is simple: Inhale deeply through the nose and exhale through the mouth nine times. When exhaling, make the sound hoo. This method of breathing will clear the lungs and throat of any obstructions, relax the entire body, and help focus and calm the mind.

For the second part, use the right index finger to close off the right nostril and breathe in through the left nostril. To exhale close off the left nostril with the left index finger and breathe through the right nostril. Do this slowly, feeling the breath expanding and contracting in the lower abdomen. Repeat the process a total of nine times.

Natural Breathing

During the meditation on the Original Cavity the breathing is initially conducted through what is called Natural Breathing. This means that the lower abdomen is expanded on the inhalation and contracted on the exhalation. Also, on the inhalation you should perform a slight drawing in and up of the anal muscles, releasing them during exhalation. The tongue must be kept on the roof of the mouth, which serves two important functions: connecting and completing the circuit of the Jenmo meridian and increasing saliva production so that the throat does not become dry and continues to nourish the body.

The methods described previously for Opening the Original should be practiced daily until you experience either flashes of light within the Original Cavity or a movement of qi within the meridians. At this point the techniques of Tortoise Breathing and Immortal Breathing should be practiced.

Tortoise Breathing

Tortoise Breathing is a method of holding the breath for long periods of time in order to efficiently move the qi through the meridians.

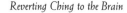

In practice one should first use mediation to learn to exhale the breath that was gathered in the lower abdomen to a count of twelve, attempting to coordinate the breath with the heartbeat. When this action becomes easy move on to exhaling to a count of thirty-six, and then finally to a count of sixty. Once you have accomplished exhaling to a count of sixty, move on to holding the inhalation for sixty counts before exhaling. If you can do this repeatedly during meditation without any strain or discomfort, you have completed the "minor tour." Taoists then seek the "middle tour" of 360 counts, and finally the "major tour" of 1,200 counts.

Immortal Breathing

Immortal Breathing really is not breathing at all, at least not in the normal sense of the word. When the practitioner reaches a heightened state in his meditation practice, breath and qi will naturally move from the soles of the feet (*yung chuan*, or Bubbling Spring cavities) through the meridians up into the brain (*t'ien ku*, or Heavenly Valley cavity).

Immortal Breathing is sometimes referred to as True Breath because it is purely internal breathing; there is no physical sensation of breath. When first experiencing True Breath many practitioners become extremely frightened when they become conscious that they are not breathing normally. It's as if everything is perfectly still, except the qi circulating throughout the meridians of the body. This type of breath is very similar to the experience of an infant in its mother's womb, surrounded by water with the lungs filled with fluids. When the baby is born the fluids drain from the lungs and it begins taking in air. This change in method of breathing must also be a frightening experience.

Achieving Immortal Breathing can take years of practice and dedication to meditation, and the only way to accomplish it is to first discipline yourself to the Natural and Tortoise Breathing methods.

SIX

The Teachings of Taoist Master Yang Chu

> *To chatter about the Tao, to gossip about the Way, none of it makes any sense.*
>
> *Heaven, earth, humanity, and me, each has its own idea for living with the Tao.*
>
> **—White Tigress Manual**

In the Taoist classic *The Book of Lieh Tzu*, which appeared sometime between 600 B.C.E. and 400 B.C.E., is a chapter dedicated to the teachings of the Taoist master Yang Chu. This teacher and his chapter, which Lieh Tzu found fit for inclusion in his book, has been the source of a great deal of controversy—mainly because it is so unlike the rest of Lieh Tzu's writing. Many have claimed that Yang Chu is no more than a hedonist, an Epicurean, and an egotistical philosopher. This view of him might be accurate if his philosophy is taken in the literal sense, as many scholars have done in the past.

Taoist philosophy should rarely be taken literally; rather, the philosophies are analogies steeped in mythical thought. Taoism is mysticism at its core, and if we look at Yang Chu's work in the light of mystical thought, we see something far beyond what his critics have claimed of him.

Yang Chu's philosophy has long been a philosophical base for both the White Tigress and the Jade Dragon practices. In the *White Tigress Manual* it occupies the very front of the work. It took me some time to understand this, but the more I looked at his work, it became abundantly clear why it is positioned so prominently in the manual.

First, Yang Chu strikes a chord with his disdain for people who live under the pretense of reputation, morality, success, and sacrifice. It is precisely these types of people who cannot, because of their fanaticism and fears, accept teachings such as those contained in the *White Tigress Manual*. But keep in mind that Yang Chu never claims that reputation, morality, success, and sacrifice are wrong. His point is that seeking them at the expense of harming yourself or living under the pretense of having achieved them is both naturally and spiritually wrong.

For example, Yang Chu states that what all people instinctively desire is good food, good music, fine clothes, and to be in the company of beautiful people of the opposite sex. But nowhere in his writings does he claim that others are to be used, deceived, manipulated, and so on in order to realize those desires. Rather, Yang Chu believes that if a person can enjoy one or all of these experiences, he should. Yang Chu preaches a philosophy of neither seeking wealth and fame nor avoiding it if shows up at your front door. To Yang Chu life is short and it should lived to its fullest. Some people are born very poor and some born very rich, but in each case one should live his life with as much joy and happiness as possible.

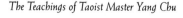

Yang Chu is expressing the same idea, with different words, of the Zen philosophy of "here and now." He objects strongly to the interference of other people, religions, and governments in the life of a person who wishes to do as he pleases—even if it seems harmful in the minds or precepts of those others. Rather, each person should live as he chooses. Likewise, people only harm themselves through the conformity of "acceptable" lifestyles and thought. This philosophy is not egotistical. In fact, it is more Taoist than most Taoists would ever envision, as Yang Chu goes to the heart of the Taoist ideals of nonconformity and noninterference.

If nothing else, Yang Chu is being honest to a fault. No one can deny his instincts for happiness and comfort. Whether we seek to drink our way to happiness or sit in joyous tranquil meditation, we are attempting to find that state of mind in which the suffering of life is ended. Yang Chu is simply stating that if one chooses to drink his way to heaven or meditate his way there, it is not anyone else's concern.

Yang Chu understood that moral beliefs are very subjective and that being moral, as a religion would define it, could never ensure a lifetime of happiness and contentment. Indeed, he sees morality as turning in and on itself. Just as Lao Tzu believed, if one expresses strong opinions of righteousness, the righteousness will become unrighteousness; those who preach morality usually end up committing immoral acts. Yang Chu is not instructing us to be immoral; he is saying that we should keep our opinions to ourselves, be good people without demanding the same of others, and be kind to others without demanding they return it to us. We should just live, find joy where we can, and not interfere with the affairs of others.

The above summary encapsulates Yang Chu's beliefs and

demonstrates why his philosophy is so attractive to the White Tigress and Jade Dragon—as it should be to all those inclined to Taoist thought.

As with most Taoist works, taking in the full import of Yang Chu's philosophy is much like an ant attempting to eat an entire watermelon with one bite. Realizing that the fifteen small sections of this chapter are full of meaning and in some cases go well beyond the intent of this book, it is important for the reader to gain the more philosophical Taoist mindset of a traditional Jade Dragon, rather than just learning the physical techniques of the sexual practices. Yang Chu's words embody an obvious celebration of freedom and naturalness as well as living fully, guided by one's own senses, rather than feeling it necessary to hang on to the social and moral dictates of society. In the end, Yang Chu affirms the value of living and being alive. Without question his philosophy was way ahead of its time. Surely he would have been quite comfortable if he had lived in our present times, especially during the sexual revolution and the hippie movement. I advise you to simply read the following chapter and allow Yang Chu's words to play about in your mind.

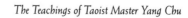

PART I
The Pretense of Reputation

One time, Yang Chu traveled to an area called Lu where he stayed with the Meng family. Master Meng put the following question to Yang Chu, "Is it not enough just to be a common person? Is it really necessary to trouble yourself with seeking fame?"

"Fame," said Yang Chu, "brings fortune."

"And then?" asked Master Meng.

"Then comes nobility," answered Yang Chu.

"And then?" asked Master Meng.

"Then comes death," responded Yang Chu.

"So one troubles himself his whole life for reputation and then just dies?" queried Master Meng.

"No, not at all," said Yang Chu. "Your reputation can be transmitted to your descendants after your death."

Master Meng then asked, "Is it absolutely certain the descendants will inherit that reputation?"

Yang Chu replied, "Indeed, the struggle of seeking a reputation does injure the body and wither the heart, but on the other hand to take advantage of a natural destiny of fame can bring prosperity to your entire clan, to the people of your district, and to all your descendants. But those who seek fame must be honest, even though honesty does not bring wealth. They must be humble, even though being humble does not bring nobility.

"For example, when Kuan Chung was the minister of Ch'i he imitated his ruler to the point that when the ruler was lewd, he was lewd; when his ruler was extravagant, he was extravagant. He served his ruler with such humility in thought and speech that through his practice of this Way (Tao) the kingdom gained great prominence and influence. But after his death, he left his family nothing.

"Then there was T'ien Heng, who was also a chief minister of Ch'i. When his ruler acted arrogant, he acted unassuming; when his ruler was miserly, he was generous. In each situation he acted the opposite of his ruler and all the people sided with him. In the end he inherited the State of Ch'i, and his descendants benefit from it to this day."

Master Meng concluded from this, "Living up to one's reputation [as did Kuan Chung] brings poverty; but if you maintain the pretense of reputation [as did T'ien Heng] you will gain wealth."

Yang Chu responded, "In these two cases it shows that reputation has little to do with reality and truth, and that truth and reality have little to do with reputation. Reputation is more often than not just a pretense. Yao and Shun were glorified because they maintained the pretense of abdicating the throne to Hsu Yu and Shan Chuan, but in reality they never gave it up because they continued to enjoy imperial favors for a hundred years. But Po Yi and Shu Ch'i, who truly resigned out of loyalty to their ideals, lost their fiefs of Ku Chu and died of starvation on Mount Shou Yang. As a result they were mourned by some, mocked by many, and

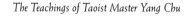

held in esteem by no one. Cannot the differences here between true reputation and pretense of reputation be clearly distinguished?"

PART II
The Pretense of Conformity

Yang Chu said, "A hundred years is considered the apex of longevity, but rarely does one man live to a hundred years of age. Assuming a man does live a hundred years or more, the great part of his life is spent in the weakness of infancy, and even a greater part in decrepitude and senility. A good portion is also taken up by the time spent in sleep and the distractions of daily living. Then there is all the time taken by pain and illness, sorrow and toil, gain and loss, and stress and fear. Of those few dozen or so years that remain, how much of that time are we really at ease and content—without anxiety? Not even the space of one hour.

"What, then, does a person live for? Where can he find happiness? Would it be in fine clothes, good food, music, and beautiful women [or men]? Even though we periodically lose our satisfactions derived from fine clothes and good food, we cannot constantly listen to music and play with women [or men]. Likewise, we are obstructed by the law and seduced by the rewards of following it, motivated by the dream of the rewards of a good reputation yet made fearful by rules of morality. Frantically we compete for even an hour of what turns out to be empty praise, and spend a lifetime scheming for a reputation that will outlive our own death. Even if in solitude we still conform to what others do, still listen to what others say, and still feel guilty about what we think—whether these thoughts are good or bad. We fail to enjoy to the utmost the prime of our lives; we fail to live in the moment. Tell me, then, how are we different from a person shackled in a prison?

"The ancients knew that life and death alternate, as we are living for but a moment and are in death for but a moment. Therefore, they did as their hearts prompted and did not reject the spontaneity of action. During their lives they did not reject the pleasures of life and sought not the seduction of fame or reputation. They roamed as they pleased and did not suppress their natural desires. Since they did not yearn for reputation that lasted after death, punishments did not affect their lives. Whether blamed or praised, whether living a long or short time, they paid no mind. They simply lived out their natures and enjoyed their lives and let others do the same."

PART III
The Equality of Death

Yang Chu said, "Each person differs in life, but not in death. Some beings are wise and others foolish, some are noble and others common—these are some of the differences. In death, however, we all are a mass of putrefied flesh; we decay and are extinguished. In this we are all the same.

"However, whether a person is wise or foolish, noble or common, is a matter of fate, just as becoming putrefied flesh, decaying, and extinguishing are not our own doing and are the same for everyone. We do not bring about either our own lives or deaths, wisdom or foolishness, nobility or commonness; all are but chance qualities shared among all people. All things live and die, are equally wise and foolish, and are equally noble and common.

"Whether in ten years or a hundred years, we all die. The saintly and wise die, the evil and foolish die. Concerning the deaths of the noble Yao and Shun and of the tyrants Chieh and Chou, all that remains is their putrefied corpses. Rotting bones are all the same; who can distinguish one from the other? Therefore, you should seek to enjoy your life while it is with you. Why bother yourself with things after death?"

PART IV
The Pretense of Pride

Yang Chu said, "It was from excessiveness of loyalty that Po Yi allowed himself to starve to death. He was not without passion, but had too much false pride about being pure. It was from excessiveness of continence that Chan Ch'in made his line extinct. He was not without passion, but had too much false pride in his morality. Because they went to these extremes, even these best of men mistakenly took purity and morality for being virtuous."

Yang Chu said, "[Of the two disciples of Confucius], Yuan Hsien of Lu was poor and Tzu Kung of Wei was wealthy. Yuan Hsien's poverty shortened his life, while Tzu Kung's wealth caused him a great deal of trouble. In light of these two examples we must ask, 'If both poverty and wealth are equally harmful, what is the right course to live by? The right course is found in simply enjoying your life and freeing yourself from worry. If you are good at enjoying your life then you are not poor, and if you are good at freeing yourself from worry then you do not care about the toils of being wealthy.'"

Yang Chu added, "There is an old saying that reads, 'Help the living and forget the dead.' This saying is absolutely correct. To help the living does not mean to simply feel sorry for them; when they are suffering we can give them comfort, if they are hungry we can feed them, if they are cold we can warm them, if they are in trouble we can go to their aid. To abandon the dead does not mean we no longer remember or feel sorry for them, but we should not be wasteful by placing pearls or jades in their mouths, dress them in rich brocades, place sacrificial victims with them, or place funereal vessels of offerings with them."

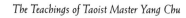

PART V
Nourishing Life

Yen Tzu asked Kuan Chung about Nourishing Life. He answered by saying, "Simply live without restraints, without suppressing natural tendencies, and without restricting yourself."

Yen Tzu requested, "Please explain more about this."

Kuan Chung continued, "Do not constrain your natural tendencies. Engage in whatever your ears wish to listen to, your eyes wish to gaze upon, your mouth wishes to speak of, your body wishes to find comfort in, or your mind wishes to find repose in. If the ears wish to hear beautiful music, then do not deny yourself; otherwise this is called constraining the sense of hearing. If the eyes wish to gaze upon beautiful women [or men], do not deny yourself; otherwise this is called constraining the sense of sight. If the nose wishes to smell orchids and spices, do not deny yourself; otherwise this is called constraining the sense of smell. If the mouth wishes to speak of truth and falsehood, then do not deny yourself; otherwise this is called constraining the sense of intelligence. If the body wishes to find comfort in wearing fine clothes and eating good food, then do not deny yourself; otherwise this is called constraining the sense of comfort. If the mind wishes to experience freedom and leisure, then do not deny yourself; otherwise this is called constraining your true nature.

"All these constraints become your masters. Rid yourself of

these oppressive masters and live unaffected by thoughts of death. Whether you live one day, one month, one year, or ten years, you will do what I call Nourishing Life. But if you attach yourself to these oppressive masters you will be unable to escape their grasp. Therefore, if you live in misery for a hundred years, a thousand years, or even ten thousand years, I would not say your were Nourishing Life."

Kuan Chung then turned a question to Yen Tzu. "I have spoken to you about Nourishing Life. Now what can you tell me how we should treat the dead?"

Yen Tzu said, "It is of no concern how we treat the dead. There really is nothing to say about this."

Kuan Chung pressed, "I insist on hearing your views."

Yen Tzu replied, "Once I am dead, I will have no more concerns. It will be of no difference to me whether you cremate me or drop my body in a river, bury me or just lay me on the open ground, wrap me in grass and toss me in a ditch or place me in a stone coffin dressed in a dragon coat and embroidered skirt. It will all be the same to me."

Kuan Chung turned and looked at his friends, Pao Shu-ya and Huang Tzu, who were listening, and said, "Both of us have said all there is to say about the Tao of living and dying."

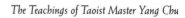

PART VI
Live and Let Live

Tzu Ch'an served as prime minister in the principality of Cheng. Within just three years he had taken charge of the entire government. His innovations and reforms proved beneficial to good people, but his prohibitions made many aristocrats discontent. But in general he brought the state into good order, and other states feared attacking it.

Tzu Ch'an had two brothers—the elder brother was Kung Sun-ch'ao and the younger brother was Kung Sun-mu. Ch'ao was very fond of wine and Mu was very fond of women. Chao had stored more than a thousand jars of wine and a mass of yeast for brewing. Within a hundred paces of his door, people could smell the odor of his wine and dregs. Ch'ao loved wine so much that he was oblivious to all worldly concerns and often lost all sense of decency and prudence. Even the possessions of his home were of no concern to him, as were his relationships with kinsmen. It was said that even if he were standing in water or fire with a sword slashing about him, he would have been totally unaware of it.

Mu had at his home a back courtyard with several dozens rooms. He selected as many lovely young girls as he could find to fill these rooms for his harem. When wanting to satisfy his desires he would shut the doors on all kinsmen and friends and would escape to his harem. The nights felt too short to him and he

 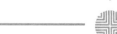

would become agitated if he was forced to leave his women once in three months. All the attractive young virgins in his district he seduced and tempted with gifts, and he would often use a go-between to help him entice women, rarely giving up on any beautiful girl he desired.

Tzu Ch'an was mortified of and very concerned about the ill conduct of his two brothers. Eventually he went to request private consul from Teng Hsi.

Tzu Ch'an said to him, "I have heard it said that men should regulate their own family by setting good examples, and regulate the state through the good examples of their family—meaning, of course, that if you pay attention to what is near you it will influence what is far from you. The government I run is in good order, but my family is in anarchy. Tell me, have I been doing things backward and wrong? Please tell me how to help my two brothers."

Teng Hsi replied, "I have long been curious of your situation but did not wish to interfere. You must look for an opportunity to help them redirect their lives, help them understand the value of maintaining their health, and call upon their senses of propriety and duty."

Tzu Ch'an accepted Teng Hsi's advice and later found the appropriate time to visit the two brothers simultaneously. He said to them: "Wisdom and perception are what set men above birds and beasts. Wisdom and perception manifest as propriety and duty in men. If you can begin to live correctly and dutifully, a good reputation and office will surely become far from you.

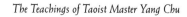

"It is knowledge, rites, and morality [Confucian ideals] that also set men above birds and beasts. Knowledge, rites, and morality are what manifest propriety and duty in men. If you can begin to live correctly and dutifully, a good reputation and office will surely become yours. But to continue simply feeding your passions and exciting yourselves with pleasure and lust, both your life and health will surely be severely injured. If you can listen to what I am telling you, repent and reform this morning. You will be able to receive your stipends by evening."

Chao and Mu responded, "For a very long time we have known what you are telling us, and many years ago we already decided on the way in which we wish to live. Why do you think your advice now will make us see something different? Life is a gift and death takes it away all too soon. This life we live is so precious, we must not forget that death will come quickly. Now you come to us and wish to impress us with your high regard for propriety and duty, clouding your natural temperament just to get a good name for yourself. In our view this is worse than death itself.

"All we wish to do is enjoy this solitude to the fullest, experiencing the most pleasure we can from our vital years. Misfortune to us is having a weak stomach that cannot endure large quantities of wine or a sexual potency that cannot be satisfied. Simply put, we have no time in which to worry and fret over reputation and ill health.

"Besides, are you not just being mean-spirited and pitiful by acting so proud of your achievements in ruling the state? Why do you come to disturb our minds with these erroneous high ideals and attempt to infect us with your grandiose thoughts of fame and profit?

"It is now our turn to debate this issue with you. A man who professes to be good at regulating the lives of others rarely succeeds at anything other than overworking and messing up his own life. But a man who is good at regulating his own life can perceive his own true nature without interfering in the lives of others. Therefore, your way of regulating others might work for ruling a state, but is out of sync with what lies in others' hearts. On the other hand, our way of regulating ourselves can be applied to everyone and can bring an end to this Tao of a ruler and those who serve him. For so long we attempted by example to help you understand our way of living, instead you just come here to preach your way to us."

Tzu Ch'an was totally dumbfounded by their reply and could think of nothing to say in response. Later, when he told Teng Hsi of this conversation, Teng Hsi replied, "Without your being aware of it, you have been dwelling with True Men. How can others say you are a sage man? Your good governing of Cheng happened by mere haphazard; there is no credit to be assigned to you for this."

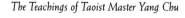

PART VII
Living As You Will

Tuan Mu-shu of Wei was a descendant of the great disciple of Confucius, Tzu Kung. He lived very opulently off his huge ancestral inheritance, providing himself and others with great pleasures and comforts. His home, gardens, food, clothing, music, and harem equaled that of the princes of Chi and Chu.

When guests visited him he would provide them with whatever they needed, even if it meant acquiring items from distant lands. When he traveled he went where he pleased and all luxuries were brought with him. Visitors flocked to him by the hundreds. He never closed his kitchens, and musicians in his court never stopped playing. He distributed his wealth generously among everyone, and he maintained this practice for sixty years. When he felt that death was near and his vitality was leaving him, all his possessions were given out as presents. But he left nothing to his children.

Tuan Mu-shu emptied his storehouses and treasuries so completely that during his final illness he had not enough money to buy the proper medicines for himself or even for his burial. But those who had received gifts from him pooled together the resources for giving him a proper funeral and restored the wealth back to his children.

When Ch'in Ku-li heard of this man and his behavior, he commented, "Tuan Mu-shu was insane and completely dishonored and disgraced his ancestor Tzu Kung." But upon hearing this Tuan Kan-sheng claimed, "Tuan Mu-shu was a superior man, surpassing his ancestor Tzu Kung in both spiritual wisdom and his economical conduct. Acting contrary to the norm of what others consider common sense, he acted on a superior sense in conforming to his true nature and temperament. Other men only conformed to what they had been taught, but he was far wiser than all the princes of Wei who criticized him."

PART VIII
Let Life Run Its Course

Meng Sun-yang asked Yang Chu, "If a person were to carefully guide his life and discipline his body, could he expect to find the way in which to live forever?" Yang Chu responded, "Such a person could live longer, but would all this effort and toil really be worth it just to add a few years to his life? A person is full of passions, dislikes and likes. It has always been this way and always will be. A person is always concerned over the health of his body, about the joy and sadness of worldly matters, about making fortunes or being poor, about the ideals of good government. It has always been this way and always will be. There is really nothing we haven't heard, seen, or experienced already. Things appear to change, but actually they are the same. So even if a person could live a hundred years or more, nothing can completely satisfy him.

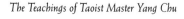

And if he did not die from sadness, boredom would surely cause his demise. Why should we undertake the toil of lengthening our lives?"

Meng then said, "If I understand you correctly, the ideal is to just end life as soon as we feel old age approaching?" Yang Chu replied, "No, that is not it at all. You should just live to the fullest while you are alive, experiencing all the satisfaction life offers while you can. When it is time to die, die. Accept and cherish the fact that life will come to an end. True living is a matter of not toiling yourself to prolong life and likewise not attempting to hasten death either."

PART IX
Not One Hair

Yang Chu said, "Po Cheng Tzu-kao claimed he would not sacrifice one hair off his body for the love of anything. Leaving the capital, he retired to plough his fields. Contrarily, the Great Yu sacrificed himself by working hard for others. While aiding in the work of draining flood waters, he worked so hard that one side of his body became paralyzed.

"Those of ancient times would not have given even one of their hairs to the empire, seeing no reason for devotion to it. Likewise, if everything in the empire were offered solely to one of them, he would not have accepted it. In those times no one saw reason to give the empire even one hair and no one wanted benefit from the empire either. This is when the empire was in good order."

Ch'in Ku-li, on hearing this from Yang Chu, asked, "But would you personally sacrifice a hair off your body for the empire?"

Yang Chu replied, "One hair would certainly not provide any benefit to the empire."

Ch'in Ku-li asked, "But if it could benefit the empire, would you?"

Yang Chu sat silently, not answering him.

Later Ch'in Ku-li was talking with Meng Sun-yang and told him of this conversation. Meng Sun-yang replied, "I do not think that you understood what my master was thinking. I will try and explain it to you. Suppose you were to be given ten thousand pieces of gold for just a small piece of your flesh and skin. Would you give it?"

"Of course I would," said Ch'in Ku-li.

Meng Sun-yang continued, "Okay, now let's suppose you would be given an entire empire of your own by severing a limb from your body, would you do so?"

Ch'in Ku-li fell silent and so Meng Sun-yang spoke. "It seems obvious that one hair is but a trifle if compared to that of a piece of flesh and skin," he said, "likewise a piece of flesh and skin is a trifle compared to a whole limb of the body. However, many hairs of the body would be equal to that of one small piece of flesh and skin, a big piece of flesh and skin would be equal to that of an entire limb. How can you think that one single hair is not as integral to the body as is a limb? How can you not see them as equally precious?"

Ch'in Ku-li said, "I really do not know how to answer this. All I know is that if this proposition was made to Lao Tzu or Kuan Yin Tzu, they would wholeheartedly agree with you. Yet if I were to present this question to the Great Yu and Mo Tzu, they would certainly agree with me."

Meng Sun-yang then turned away, ignoring Ch'in Ku-li, and changed the subject with his disciples, who were sitting there listening.

PART X
The Vexation of Propriety and Duty

Yang Chu said, "Everyone speaks admirably of Shun, Yu, the Duke of Chou, and Confucius, and yet everyone condemns Chieh and Chou.

"Shun worked hard as a farmer in Ho-yang and made pottery in Lei-tse. He never gave his body any comfort or rest, never ate good food, was unloved by his parents, and was shunned by his brothers and sisters. He did not marry until he was thirty, and then did so without receiving permission from his parents. When Yao abdicated his throne he handed the empire over to Shun, but Shun was already old and his mind was waning. Shun's eldest son, Shang Chun, was completely incompetent, so Shun had to turn over the throne to Yu instead of his son. Shun lived morosely in old age and died a miserable death, something all men of the Way try to avoid.

"When Kun, the father of Yu, attempted to drain the water that flooded the empire, he failed. Shun had him executed in Yu Shan. Yu took over his father's work and so served the very person responsible for his father's death, but his only concern was serving his empire. Yu's children and property were neglected, he was too busy to visit his own house, one side of his body was paralyzed from too much work, and his hands and feet were raw and bent from the calluses. When Shun gave the throne to Yu, the palace was maintained meagerly; only Yu's sash and cap had any elegance about them. He also died a miserable death, and his life was filled with excessive worry and responsibility.

"After King Wu died but during the youth of Emperor Cheng, the Duke of Chou was placed in charge of the empire. But the Duke of Shao was displeased with this decision and went about spreading rumors to injure the Duke of Chou, which resulted in the Duke of Chou resigning and going into exile for three years. His elder brother was executed and his younger brothers were banished. The Duke of Chou himself barely escaped with his own life. He also died a miserable death, and his whole life seemed to be filled with nothing but danger and fear.

"Confucius spent most of his life extolling the merits of the old emperors, accepting invitations from the princes of his time so he could propagate his teachings. But in return for all his efforts they felled a tree over his shelter in Sung, evicted him from Wei, drove

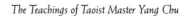

him to poverty in Sung and Chou, and trapped him with a blockade in Ch'en and Ts'ai. He was provoked and humiliated by the Ch'i family and outrageously insulted by Yang Hu. He suffered a miserable death, and his entire life was filled with agitation and distress.

"All four of these great sages lived without one day of joy and contentment, yet their reputations will live on for ten thousand years. The truth and reality of all their efforts amounted to no more than a vain posthumous reputation; this was their only reward for a whole life deprived of pleasure. Even though today we praise them and make offerings to them, they know nothing of it; even though we honor them, they know nothing of it. All this praise and honor is as worthless to them as a rotted tree stump or clump of dirt is to us.

"Conversely, Chieh, who inherited all the riches and powers from successive emperors, enjoyed all pleasures during his time on the throne. He satisfied all his appetites, was witty enough to keep all his subjects in servitude, and made everyone as far as the four seas tremble with his authoritative manner. He amused his eyes and ears with complete abandon, and whatever his thoughts and inclinations were he acted on them. Up to his death he led a very free, happy, and boisterous life.

"Chou also inherited all the riches and powers from successive reigns, and during his time on the throne he rejected the ceremonial rites and exerted his authority throughout the empire. Within his hundred-acre palace he satisfied all his passions, hosting banquets that would last four months but treating them as if they were single nights. During his reign he never worried about matters of propriety and duty. He died by execution, but he led a very carefree, happy, and unconstrained life.

"These two men lived life to the fullest. But now the people consider them ignorant and immoral fools. But these views mean nothing to them now, and they have no knowledge of what others think of them. All of it, whether praise or blame, means no more to them then a rotted tree stump or clump of dirt.

"The four sages, even though praised and revered to this day, lived in endless suffering and died pitifully, with their only reward for all this sacrifice being a vain and meaningless reputation. In the end death was their last dwelling place. But the so-called ignorant and immoral fools, even though they are blamed and condemned to this day, enjoyed their lives to the fullest, and death was also their last dwelling place."

PART XI
Instructing an Emperor

Once Yang Chu met with the Emperor of Liang. During this meeting he told the emperor that governing an empire was no more difficult than simply turning over one's hand. The emperor responded, "Master, you have both a wife and a concubine, both of which you cannot control. You also have a three-acre garden you cannot properly tend. Yet you dare advise me that ruling an empire is as easy as turning over my hand. Are you attempting to make fun of me?"

Yang Chu then said, "Have you ever seen a shepherd leading his flock? Even a boy four feet tall, with just a staff on his shoulder, can lead the sheep in any direction he chooses. But if we take the example of Yao pulling in front and Shun pushing from behind, they couldn't make even one of the sheep budge. In regard to my affairs, which you made notice of, I can only tell you this: Fish that are big enough to swallow a boat do not attempt to swim in small streams, and hawks and swans do not rest in puddles. Why? Because their instincts and natures are far beyond it. The music of Huang-chung and Ta-lü are not fitting for dancers. Why? Because it is far beyond the ordinary form of music. Therefore it is said that those who are capable of managing great affairs do not fret over trifles. Those who accomplish great success do not seek to accomplish small success. I think you now understand my meaning."

PART XII
The Impermanence of Reputation

Yang Chu said, "The myriad events of antiquity have vanished; we cannot remember but a few. The doings of the Three August Ones are also almost completely lost. The actions of the Five Sovereigns are muddled like a dream. Of the affairs of the Three

Emperors, we remember not even a thousandth of them. Even in present times, of all events we can remember barely one in a thousand. When it comes to current events, we see some and ignore others but we cannot remember but one in a thousand. The years and events starting in antiquity to the present day are just too numerous for anyone to record in memory.

"In the three thousand years since the time of Fu-hsi and the thousands of years preceding him, there have been men of wisdom, men of ignorance, beautiful and ugly things, successes and failures, and good and evil. All of them have faded in human memory; the constant is that they all fade, whether slowly or quickly.

"If we rule our lives with thoughts of praise and blame for even an hour, all we accomplish is destroying our spirits and injuring our bodies—all just to gain a reputation that could at best last a few hundred years after our deaths. The effort of gaining reputation costs a lifetime of denying the pleasures of life. How will this moisten our dried bones and bring back the joy of being alive after our deaths?"

PART XIII
The Intelligence of Humans

Yang Chu said, "The human being is really no different than all other species within nature; all owe their existence to the workings of the Five Elements. But of all living things, the human being is

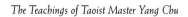

the most intelligent. Yet the human has not teeth and claws strong enough to provide adequate defense, skin impenetrable enough for adequate protection, feet and legs agile or fast enough to escape danger, and adequate fur or hair for protection from heat and cold. The human survives off the subsistence of other creatures and things, which he completely dominates, primarily doing so through intelligence rather than force. It is the human's intelligence that makes him superior to all the other creatures, even though many other creatures are far stronger than the human.

"My physical body is really not my possession alone, but since my birth I have had no option but to maintain it. All other creatures and things are likewise not my possession, yet to exist I have no option but to make use of them. I am alive because of my body, yet it is only through other things that I can keep my body alive. But even though I keep my body alive, I cannot truly possess either it or my life. I may make use of other creatures and things to stay alive, yet I cannot truly possess any of them.

"It is not possible for a human to give himself life, and other species cannot give themselves life either. Therefore, a sage person does not treat any life form that nourishes his life lightly, regarding all things as equal and superior. This is why it is said that the sage is the highest and most superior of all beings."

PART XIV
The Ideal of Indifference

Yang Chu said, "There are four desires that plague all people. They are the desire for longevity, the desire for reputation, the desire for position, and the desire for wealth. Those who manage to acquire these four desires live in fear of losing them. They fear both the living and the dead, and they fear others in authority and the punishments that could be inflicted on them. Living in constant fear, they do not know anything of destiny and fate; they erroneously believe that external circumstances are what control their lives. Sadly, their whole lives are lived in flight from their fears.

"But there are people who just live by their destiny and accept what fate brings them; they do not bother themselves with thoughts of longevity, reputation, positions, and wealth. Since they do not oppose destiny, they accept whatever life span is given to them. Since they are not arrogant about being praised, they do not worry about reputation. Since they are not concerned about having power, they do not seek position. Since they are not affected by greed, wealth does not concern them. These are people who live in harmony with destiny.

"It is said that the desire for love causes half of a person's troubles in life, and the desire for comfort causes the rest. Another proverb from the Chou dynasty says, 'It is easier to hunt pheasants if you simply wait for them to sit upon the ground.'

"A simple farmer might well be the happiest person on Earth because working a whole day feels natural and normal to him. He finds satisfaction in eating the food he has grown, and his skin and muscles are strong and vigorous. If he was to lie upon soft furs while draped in fine silks and was given delicacies to eat, he would fall ill and break into a fever. Yet if an emperor were to change places with a farmer, he would fall exhausted even after an hour's work. Therefore, when a common laborer is satisfied with the fruits of his labor, he thinks nothing in the world could be better.

"In the Sung dynasty there was a farmer who wore a tattered hemp coat, which barely kept him from the cold of winter. In the spring he would go about naked, warming his body in the sunshine. Having no concept of palaces with rooms laden with furs and silks, he told his wife, 'The emperor should know of this. I am sure he will reward me if I tell him the great comfort of being naked in the warm sun.'

"A rich man in his village overheard this and advised the farmer, 'Once a peasant offered some simple food items to the prince of his district. But when he ate the peasant's food it caused him stomach pains and a bad taste in his mouth. For this the peasant was mocked and sent away in shame. You are now thinking of repeating the same error. The emperor cannot learn your secret of warming the naked body in the sun.'"

PART XV
Do Not Seek or Avoid

Yang Chu said, "A good house, fine clothing, good food, and beautiful women [or men]. Having these, what more could a person really want? Those who seek more than these are insatiable, and these people only injure their lives and wear out their bodies, becoming like a piece of worm-eaten wood. Between their egos and their discontentment, they do not respect their rulers or others. When they appear to be respectful of others it is only out of desire to advance themselves.

"The Way of the ancients was to be in harmony and at peace with everyone. Yu Tzu said, 'Get rid of the desire for reputation and life will be without disappointments.' Lao Tzu said, 'Reputation is not equal to knowing the truth of things, yet people will chase after reputation before seeking the truth.'

"Reputation should not be sought nor avoided. The efforts of seeking reputation only bring injury, but its natural occurrence brings great comfort. To experience dishonor by failing to achieve reputation brings great sadness and suffering. Do not seek a fabricated reputation, but accept it if destiny provides it. The ideal is to have indifference toward acquiring or losing reputation."

SEVEN

The Bamboo Immortal

(The Jade Dragon Li Huang)

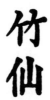

> *The Tao of all the immortals and immortalesses,*
> *first lies in the accumulation and refinement of the ching;*
> *then the ch'i can be transmuted so it ascends,*
> *uniting with and illuminating the shen.*
> *Thus, the Yellow Stream opens the gateway to perfect bliss.*
>
> **—White Tigress Manual**

This chapter contains a translation of the biographical record of Taoist master Li Huang (1712–?). During his lifelong pursuit of Taoism he became a Jade Dragon with one of Chin Hua's students (Chin Hua was the first White Tigress to begin compiling the *White Tigress Manual* in 1748). At her request, he wrote a brief record of his experiences of being a Taoist, a Jade Dragon, and later a Taoist hermit.

In many ways this record serves as a guide for present-day Taoist enthusiasts, as it clearly shows the life and practice transitions he had to make in order to delve so deeply into Taoism. It also shows what is possible for any man who sincerely embarks on the Way.

And it is also a very interesting story. Taoist literature is filled with mystical writings meant for teaching adepts; it is rare to find pieces written on a personal basis, and here Li Huang touches deeply on his personal life as a Taoist monk.

Prologue

This is my, Li Huang's, personal record, revealing my involvement, experiences, and minor spiritual accomplishments within the practices and teachings of the Taoist sects of Cheng-I and Green Dragon–White Tiger. I was born in a southwest municipality of Nanjing during the reign of emperor K'ang Hsi of the Ching dynasty in the year 1712. Presently I am writing this record in excellent health at the august age of seventy-six. Since age 29 I have resided in this small mountain hermitage called the Azure Clouds of Tranquillity in a remote section of Lung-Hu Shan (Dragon-Tiger Mountains). There are seven highly devoted and exceptionally spiritually gifted Taoist masters, all eighty years and beyond, living in this splendid hermitage. There are also nine younger novices, whom we foresee continuing the maintenance of our tranquil abode when we all mount our dragons and cranes for an even more lofty existence within in the paradises of heavenly immortals.

Even though I cannot claim spiritual accomplishments even remotely as profound and lofty as my present elder brethren, my skill throughout my life has been the study of books and writing, due mostly to the insistence of my late father, who sacrificed so much to ensure my education. As a result, now in my august years, I wish to leave behind this record partially in dire hope that others will find some inspiration for embarking upon the Way so that they too may find tranquillity, health, and longevity, as I have had the good fortune to do. Additionally, this record fulfills a promise made long ago to the Immortaless Chin Hua, who encouraged me on more than one occasion to write an honest, detailed account of my experiences and influences that assisted in forming and refining my spiritual fetus of immortality. Therefore, with all humility I declare my words are genuine and true.

My Early Influences and Experiences

In my youth I suffered from a weak physical constitution, being frail, underweight, often very lethargic, and seeming to always contract one illness after another. My parents desperately attempted to find cures to strengthen me, but none had any lasting effect. The diagnosis was that I was born with weakened and underdeveloped kidneys, which caused frequent sharp pains and soreness in my back. The herbal and moxibustion treatments had some positive effects but were not long-lasting enough to effect a permanent cure. As one healer told my father, "Just as we cannot make a deformed limb normal, there is no way to enlarge the kidneys to normalcy either." So I was left with measures that merely alleviated the pain, but I had no cure. My life expectancy was dismal—thirty years, at best, was the standard prognosis.

My father was a merchant, somewhat successful but by no means lavishly rich, and so treatments for my condition put a great strain on family finances. My mother worried constantly that I would not live long enough to acquire a wife and produce grandchildren for her, especially a male child for the family posterity. As I was the only male child in the family, this was of the greatest concern to both my parents. When I was ten years old an arranged marriage had been agreed on with the daughter of a local family. But the family was driven into poverty because of bad business dealings and out of shame moved in stealth to another province, leaving me wifeless.

By age seventeen my condition had not really improved, and to my mother's dismay there was no interest from the other families in our community for submitting a marriage proposal to any of the available daughters. Even the go-betweens in our community put off my mother on several occasions, claiming there were no available female prospects that they felt were deserving of her son. But this was just a polite way of saying that no females were interested in me because of my debilitated condition. I would even overhear my father's two concubines, Feng Hsi and Feng Sung (twins), who were close to my own age (I was sixteen and they were seventeen when my father took them as his concubines), snickering and cruelly gossiping about me, calling me a "green cap"* and gibbering that I was so weak I would never be capable of entering a woman.

---

*In Chinese society *green cap* is a slanderous term for males who suffer from impotence or some other sexual dysfunction that makes them incapable of achieving erection. The term comes from the old Chinese myth that turtles could not have sex with each other because of their cumbersome shells or green caps. It was believed that a snake had to come along to impregnate the female turtles. Hence, a green cap was incapable of impregnating his wife and would have to rely on a surrogate male to do so.

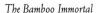

All this left me with a feeling of shame and added to my frequent inclination toward suicide. I felt it might be a better option than living in such a sickly condition all the time. But I persevered because of the love of my parents and my two younger sisters, Mei Li and Mei Hsun, who constantly pampered and cared for me and would scold and sometimes beat my father's concubines when they overheard the two girls ridicule me. The oldest of my sisters, Mei Li, who was born under the sun of the Boar, was especially loyal and quick-tempered. She was even more than my father could at times handle, and he rarely interfered with her admonishments of his concubines. She lived by a code: If someone gave her happiness she would return it threefold; if someone gave her unhappiness she would return that threefold. My father always humorously contended that the man she married better have two talents, a civil tongue and martial skills, if he expected to live a happy life with her.

My parents adhered to all three popular Chinese philosophies—Confucianism, Buddhism, and Taoism—as did many families living in our community. As a young boy, my parents always took me to the local temples for various celebrations and events. But honestly, I did not enjoy them much, as they always seemed to drain me of my energy and I often felt that I could not muster the appropriate reverence for the seemingly endless ceremonial rituals attached to these events. Add to that my distaste for having to accompany and spend any amount of time with my father's two concubines, for all I remember of them is their constant gossip and attention-getting manipulations of my father, which obviously annoyed my mother greatly. Normally on these outings I would feign some sort of malady, and my father would instantly send me home under Mei Li's care.

But on certain occasions I found myself very attracted to visiting a certain local Taoist temple on the outskirts of town. The abbot of the temple, Master Chang, was a very intriguing man, never seeming ill at ease about anything and obviously very insightful. He was always smiling and laughing, even if he was actually scolding someone. Mei Li and I usually had to be beckoned by my father to leave.

The abbot was an elderly man, but his face was very rosy and robust behind his long white beard. When walking with him it always amazed me how nimble and sprightly he was. Supposedly he had lived in a hermitage for more than sixty years on Hua Shan, but he claimed that he missed interacting with people and so he moved to and took charge of this small temple. My father told me that the abbot actually left Hua Shan because he had a nephew who in his late years grew sick, and the abbot came to Nanjing to restore his health. When the word spread of the abbot's healing skills, numerous people came to him for healing, so he was compelled to never go back to Hua Shan.

It was Master Chang who helped me recover from my weak health and guided me toward achieving immortality. On one of my visits I had offered to help tend the vegetable garden, and while I was kneeling and pulling up the many creeping weeds that

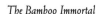

intended to choke the life from the vegetable plants, the abbot strolled by and startled me with a comment. With a broad grin on his face and in a very jovial manner he blurted out, "I think the only time you feel really alive and happy is when you come to visit us poor immortals. But what makes you happiest is when you secretly watch your sister Mei Li undress and bathe. Am I right or not?"

Dumbfounded, I could not speak. I didn't want to admit he was right about my watching my sister, which I had done frequently. So out of nervousness I said in a cracked voice, "Yes, I love coming here." But my mind raced in an attempt to figure out how he knew I had watched her, and how he knew it made me so happy. Mei Li was very beautiful, and seeing her naked body did make me feel alive. But I always assumed it was an innocent indiscretion. After a short pause and hearty chuckle he spoke again. "Mei Li knows you are watching her," he told me. "She loves you very much and hopes it will make you stronger so you will seek the amorous attention of a female. She wishes you the good fortune of obtaining a good wife and excellent children. But don't worry; this is a very natural thing between siblings. A young man's sexual curiosity is the natural means by which he is driven into manhood." Just as soon as he said that he turned and strolled lightly away, humming some poetic verse that I could not understand.

For whatever reason, I sat on my knees with tears streaming down my cheeks. My emotions were so mixed. On one hand I felt so exposed and ashamed, and couldn't figure out how Master

Chang knew this secret of mine; on the other hand I felt like I made a public admission of my fondness for my voyeuristic inclinations. Would he tell my parents? Would he tell Mei Li? Oh, the consequences raced through my mind. I was traumatized and too confused to know what to do next. Simultaneously I thought, Should I hasten to Master Chang and seek forgiveness and advice, or should I simply sneak out the temple grounds and never return? Being young, I choose the latter, returning home as quickly as I could.

For the next several days I prevented myself from thinking about what Master Chang had said and from watching my sister bathe. Instead I busied myself with reading books from my father's library. I found myself curiously drawn to such writings as *Biographies of the Immortals*, *Collected Poems of Lu Tung Pin*, *Pao P'u Tzu*, and *Lieh Tzu*. I feigned attraction to these works to my father as nothing more than a curiosity about Taoist philosophy—purely academic. But my true intent was to figure out Master Chang, for it frightened me deeply that anyone could reach into my inner mind and pull out personal actions so clearly, as though simply drawing water from a well. But alas, the books never answered my questions, at least not in a way that I could understand at the time.

Late one evening while scouring through my father's library, I happened to remove a silk-covered box from the upper shelf. Having seen it many times, I had never actually examined it because the outside of the box indicated that these were masonry texts. But on this occasion of curiosity and boredom I did remove it. Once I unfastened the ivory pegs and opened the box I saw that there were ten small scrolls. Rolling each one out, I soon discovered these were sexual manuals, describing in torrid detail how a man could utilize a woman's yin energy through "rain and clouds" methods [sexual activity] to rebuild his own yang energy, which would improve his health, longevity, and, in more serious practice, give him immortality.

I was young and curious and these texts caught my undivided attention. Each evening I would smuggle one of the scrolls back to my bedchamber and copy it by hand. Fearing my father or sisters would discover my forgery, I hid my copies in a satchel high up behind where the ceiling beams met the wall. Late each evening I would retrieve them and pore over all the instructions. This led to frequent self-abuse, as I could not help needing release as my mind wandered from one lustful thought to another.

Several weeks later I had still found convenient excuses for not returning to see Master Chang, instead distracting myself with the sex manuals. What intrigued me the most, however, was the notion that I could heal my condition through sexual means. I desperately wished I had a wife, concubine, or sexual partner to carry out the instructions. But alas, my fate was to be alone. I would have considered employing prostitutes, but that would have meant going to my father for the means to do so, and that was out of the question. He was already spending a small fortune on me for school and private tutors—proper education for his only son being his utmost priority.

To help curb my lustful demeanor I took up meditation, sitting cross-legged in my room twice a day and counting my breaths. It was for the most part a vain effort; with no formal training or teacher to guide me, I more often than not drifted into a sound, deep sleep or half-awake dream states. But I persisted as best I could, some days feeling focused and other days feeling inept enough to argue within myself about quitting altogether. I actually might have quit, except the meditation posture had a curious beneficial effect on my spine, actually giving me the sense it was strengthening my body and sometimes completely alleviated the pain in my kidneys. When time afforded itself, I would attempt to study and read the various Taoist books in my father's library in hopes of broadening my experience with meditation, but the philosophy was too difficult for me to grasp and my mental capacity for understanding the underlying mystical language was by no means adequate for the task.

During these early years I had several recurring dreams in which an unearthly beautiful female, an immortaless for certain, would appear and inform me of my destiny for immortalship. She did this while extending her hand, in which a large ripened and fragrant peach sat, and beckoning me to take it and consume it. Desperately I would attempt to reach out to seize the peach, but to no avail; my arms were rigidly frozen at my sides.

Invariably these dreams took place along a deserted, high mountainous footpath that was cut precariously along a precipice with cliffs dropping hundreds of feet below. The path was like-

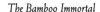

wise filled with deep and ominous black holes. My task was to follow the woman along this perilous pathway, with the promise that if I placed my feet within her footsteps I would reach safety. But always I would freeze, unable to move forward, and such panic would ensue that I would awaken myself in a cold shaking sweat.

With a sense of great shame I must confess that my fondness for peering at my sister Mei Li bathing developed eventually into actual amorous contact. I justified my bad behavior with the excuse of replenishing my yang with her yin. My ignorant adolescent mind, beset by youthful sexual impulses, devised a means whereby I could achieve contact with her and apply some of the techniques in the sex manuals without actually going so far as to engage in clouds and rain. In the back of my mind, fortunately, was the knowledge that my sister was promised in marriage, and within the year she would be moving to another prefecture to join her betrothed. I did not want her to be returned to our family in great shame for not revealing the blood of her virginity on her wedding day, so I resisted all impulses for intercourse.

Over a period of months, with her awareness of my watching her bathe and my coy signals revealing that I was watching, the activity culminated in my arranging for her to enter my room naked, pretending that it was an accident. My lower body was fully exposed, with the quilt pulled over my upper body to hide my head but not my manhood. I was pretending to be asleep for a few moments. Then I would feign a sharp pain in my back, at

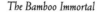

which point my sister would always come to comfort me, and I would direct her dainty hands to my swollen member.

More often than not she would gently stroke me just to the point before ejaculation, and then squeeze the base firmly and pinch the opening at the top of my penis to prevent my dissipation. Sometimes this would cause extremely ecstatic states of mind, much more intense than anything I had experienced in meditation. But my sister grew fond of watching my semen ejecting and gradually persisted each time in making me ejaculate. She justified this with the concept that her poor older brother may never enjoy the pleasures of yin and yang harmony, and so out of compassion she wanted to provide me with some experience of feeling a female's touch. She claimed that releasing my pent-up seed was both healthy and natural.

Fortunately, our encounters never went beyond touching. So despite my shame about this incestuous behavior, limited as it may have been, I confess that it gave me a profound sense of vigor that I had rarely felt before. But even more, it provided a glimpse of how powerful sexual energy could be when ejaculation was prevented.

Three months after my sister married and left our household, my father was killed by bandits, leaving me in charge of the family business. My temperament was not inclined toward business and so the company suffered greatly at my hands. Within a year my mother also died of what my youngest sister, Mei Hsun, deemed a broken heart. I was never close to my mother; I

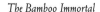

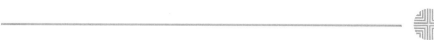

respected and honored her and she me, but there was always something missing in our relationship. Often I thought she was simply disappointed in both my frail health and me. Despite this and even though I never cried over the death of my father, whom I loved dearly, I cried and became extremely forlorn for months over my mother's death.

Within the ensuing year my younger sister had moved from the family compound to join her betrothed. I had no intentions of living at the compound with my father's concubines, whom I detested and whose constant selfish bickering and complaints about how much they suffered with my father I could not bear listening to. This talk was an erroneous attempt to affect my sympathy in order to falsely obtain whatever possessions and money they could. One evening when they finally realized I was unaffected by their false "victim" pleas, they both escaped in the darkness of night, taking with them some of my mother's jewelry and other items. I consoled myself with the happiness of never having to hear their high-pitched irritating voices again.

Staying alone in the family compound proved peaceful but also difficult. I had driven the family business to near annihilation as I attached myself to long periods of meditation every day. Eventually I had to sell the family property, and with nowhere else to go I decided to donate the proceeds from the sale to Master Chang at Heavenly Portal Temple in hopes of being allowed to take up residency there. I steadfastly decided I would become a Taoist monk and spend my days in tranquillity and detachment from the world, which up to this point in my life had shown me more loss and suffering than gain and happiness.

The Heavenly Portal Temple

Standing outside the main gate of the Heavenly Portal Temple, with just a satchel containing a few necessary personal items, I pondered what to say to Master Chang when he laid eyes on me. It had been more than two years since I scurried out from behind the temple walls on that day he revealed his knowledge of my illicit viewing of my sister Mei Li. My father had several times informed me after returning from visiting Master Chang that the abbot had inquired about my welfare. When my father would excuse me by responding that I wasn't up to traveling outside the family home, Master Chang would always make the sincere offer to help me recover if I could manage to stay with him for a few months. Partly out of shame—and because I really didn't want to leave the pleasures of Mei Li—I always found an excuse not to do so. But now life had changed so much for me, and I believed my last refuge for any happiness laid behind the austere stone walls and bright red lacquered doors of the Heavenly Portal Temple.

For so long I had envisioned myself walking into the temple and going straightaway to Master Chang to let him know that I most assuredly decided to become a Taoist monk, like a giddy child scurrying to his father with good news. I imagined he would smile broadly and exclaim his happiness, and then take me to my

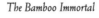

quarters to settle in for a life of tranquillity and immortality. But now that I was here, standing just two feet from the gate, I could not raise my arm to either knock or push open the door. My entire insides had frozen and a swell of remorse, fear, and sadness overcame me; never had I felt so worthless and undeserving. My satchel fell from my hands and onto my knees, and I began to cry profusely as my body trembled violently. Again I wanted to run but could not move. All I could do was remain slumped and crying.

At some point an old woman passing by saw me. She inquired as to whether or not I was okay, but I could not answer. Disappearing through the temple door, she returned quickly with a novice monk who repeatedly attempted to find out if I was okay and what I wanted of this humble temple. The only words that would leave my mouth were "tell . . . Master Chang." The novice then disappeared and the old woman leaned over next to me, placing comforting hands on my shoulders.

When the temple doors opened again, there stood in a most majestic pose Master Chang. Smiling, he reached into his robe and produced a bright yellow peach and extended it to me saying, "Follow me. Only a few simple steps and your obstacles will be broken." Picking myself up, I staggered and lunged more than walked through the gate. Once inside I felt light—lighter than I had ever felt. Master Chang turned and walked across the courtyard in a very spry gate. When he reached the other side he turned and yelled to me, "The peach is for those who find the Way. I will present it to you when the time is appropriate. For now, I suggest you rest. A humble apartment has been prepared for you; please accept our poor dwellings and honor us with your presence as long as you wish." With that he again turned and walked away with his sky blue robe fluttering as if he were about to take flight and disappeared quickly as he turned down a corridor.

His tone and demeanor were so different from what I remembered of him. He spoke as if it were the first time we ever met and appearing so bright, majestic, and stern, whereas I had remembered him as being so ordinary, carefree, and jovial. I wondered if maybe within the last two years he had achieved true immortality, and now every fiber of his being had underwent transformation. Something had to have happened because he honestly looked so much wiser, younger, and more robust.

A young novice motioned for me to follow him, so I picked up my satchel and walked silently with him until we arrived at a small building situated at the back side of the temple compound. He led me to one of ten doors, then stepped back and with three quick bows from his waist he simply smiled and said, "Welcome. I will check with you later to see if there is anything you might need to make your stay more comfortable." With that he left, and I entered the small apartment.

The room contained a small, wooden hand-carved bedchamber, intricately designed with the Eight Immortals on the upper portion of the frame. Through the sheer gauze covering the front of the bed I could see a thin wadded mat and a neatly rolled quilt and two bolsters, one which was shaped like a crescent; I assumed it was used as a meditation cushion. There were only two other items of furniture in the room: a stand with a wash basin and a hutch for storage of clothing and personal items.

The most unique part of the room, however, was a large circular window opening. The lattice design was the longevity symbol fashioned in oil-soaked rice paper, which glowed a beautiful yellow from the sunlight outside. Moving over to the window I gently swung the two partitions open to reveal a well-kept rock garden framed by dense bamboo and one juniper whose shape had been modified to look like floating clouds.

On both sides of the window were hung two beautiful scroll paintings. On the right side was the image of the Taoist immortal Lu Tung-pin, and on the left side was an excellent calligraphy piece done by the hand of Master Chang. The characters *tzu ran* (meaning "to be naturally," or "just so") written bold and large on that painting. Right below the window on a small shelf stood a tripod incense burner made of bronze with two dragons protruding from each side and acting as handles.

I sat on the edge of the bed, feeling so grateful for Master Chang's generosity in providing me with such tranquil and beautiful accommodations in which to cultivate myself. Little did I know at the time how long I would be here and what paths lay ahead of me.

As suggested by Master Chang, I rolled out the bed mat to take a rest but fell into a deep slumber, sleeping more peacefully than

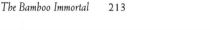

I had in years. In my dream that afternoon I remember seeing Master Chang walk by my window. He peered in with a broad smile and said, "You have finally returned now, so try your best."

Over the next four years I learned much and practiced internal alchemy and meditation exclusively, but I failed to actually form the Elixir of Immortality within myself. My life there was generally occupied with the daily duty of gardening, as I found this to be something I really enjoyed. The Heavenly Portal Temple, like most Taoist institutions, had no formalized structure; each monk mostly did what he pleased or had a talent for, as long as his activities did not disturb the other residents or bring harm to the temple. Each monk was free to pursue whatever practices, studies, or hobbies he deemed fit for his path. Since I had been able to donate a large sum of money to the coffers of the temple, I really did not have to perform any physical labor. But tending the vegetable garden and the landscape foliage made me feel good, so over time I took all that upon myself.

The temple grounds consisted of about forty acres, with the five main buildings taking up about a third of the entirely walled acreage. The layout consisted of a main stone courtyard just inside the main gate. Facing the courtyard was the main hall, which was divided into three sections: the center hall held the altar of the Three Pure Ones; to the right was an altar for Lu Tung-pin, and on the left was a most curious altar for Hsi Wang Mu and her three immortalesses. On the left side of the main hall was a long building that contained a kitchen, storage rooms, an herbal preparation room, a library, lavatories, bathing rooms, and an administration room for all the temple's affairs. The right side of the main hall was divided into two sections; on the far end were living quarters for guests, a meditation hall, an oracle room, and the patient's room, where Master Chang would administer his healing methods (including acupuncture, moxibustion, herbal remedies, and massage). Behind the main hall was a private courtyard where the monks would practice their sword exercises or kung fu practices. Behind that were two buildings set back into the tall pines, willows, and bamboo trees, and these housed the living compartments for the residents of the temple.

Besides me there were five permanent resident monks of Heavenly Portal, and at any given time three to seven novices who either came from another monastery to learn something specific from one of the teachers or were simply wandering monks needing a place to stay for a while. Of the resident monks, there is one in particular on whom I wish to comment. He had no name; we had no idea how old he was, and we had no knowledge of where he came from or was born. If you asked him what his name was, he would always respond, *"ming ke ming, fei chang ming"* ("the name that can be named is not the eternal name", this is from the first chapter of the *Tao Te Ching*). If you asked where he was born he would respond, "All things are unborn; everything comes from nothing." If you asked where he came from, he would touch you with his index and middle fingers on the shoulder and send you flying back ten feet. This man, whom we called Tao

Shih [Taoist Master], spent all his days in meditation, and on certain occasions he could be seen performing his Eight Immortal Sword Exercises or a type of fencing called Wu-T'ang Mountain Immortals' Swordplay. It was said that he only ate four times a week, supposedly living off wind and dew. Admittedly, in all my years there I rarely saw him in the dining room with the rest of us. We never had a conversation, but I felt I learned much from him.

During the first few years of my residency at Heavenly Portal Temple I did make some progress in my health and knowledge of Taoism, but I felt I was still very far away from any type of transformation to immortality. My accomplishment of sitting tranquil had improved greatly, but I had not achieved the circulation of qi through my meridians, nor had I experienced Illumination. Maybe it was impatience, maybe it was simply that I did not have the necessary temperament for the steadfast discipline of Tao Yin practices [the Taoist breathing techniques of leading and guiding the qi]. Master Chang had constantly encouraged me to continue for as long as it would take. I am sure my impatience grew thin with him, as I was constantly seeking more and more instruction from him. Somehow in the back of my mind I thought I was missing something or wasn't being told the deeper secrets, for surely I was certain that I had the intellect and desire to go much further.

But all this would change when Master Chang introduced me to a woman, Chin Hua. On previous occasions I had seen her at the temple for various festivals and meetings with Master Chang. But I always shied away from actually holding a conversation

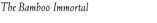

with her because she was simply too beautiful and my mind would still be distracted with thoughts of Mei Li and how incredible her touch felt. Chin Hua was even more beautiful than my sister, and for the sake of keeping my present practices intact I shunned all inclinations of drawing close to this woman.

The Immortaless Chin Hua

Early one evening as I was reading and studying my favorite Taoist work, the *Pao P'u Tzu* by the immortal Ko Hung, a light tapping was heard on my door. It was the new novice, Kuan Meng, coming to give me a message that Master Chang wished to have my presence in the garden pavilion, called Restoring Peace, near the rear of the property. It was primarily the private garden for Master Chang, where he could find and enjoy solitude from all the daily affairs of the temple. Thanking Kuan Meng, I closed my book reverently and returned it to the shelf and changed my robe and straightened my topknot and cap. I thought Master Chang was going to give me instructions to improve my meditation practice, which made me very anxious, but little was I aware of how life-changing this meeting would be.

As I approached the garden along the stone path, I overheard Master Chang laughing while a woman was speaking to him. When I made the turn around the high jagged rocks that hid the view of the small pavilion, I saw that he was sitting with the beautiful Chin Hua. Seated at a low lacquered table and on a matching stool, Master Chang caught sight of me and motioned with his hand for me to join them quickly. My apprehension grew; I feared having to sit close to her. After all, I had chosen to lead a life of celibacy and meditation, and this woman could, with one glance or brush of her delicate hand, disrupt all four years of my practice. But I had no choice. To run away would have been an enormous insult to Master Chang, so I put on my best air of ease and stepped up into the pavilion. After the pleasantries of low introductory bows, I retreated to a stool on the opposite side of the table, sitting across and as far away from Chin Hua as I could.

Master Chang offered me a small cup of the peach brandy they were drinking but I politely refused, as I never had a taste for any alcohol. (I had read accounts of the Taoist band the Seven Sages of the Bamboo Grove, who imbibed great quantities of wine before discussing the Tao and "battling" with poems throughout the night, but it had never appealed to my sensibilities.) So there I was, sitting in this beautiful garden with the most beautiful woman I had ever laid eyes on and with my most honored and revered teacher, who was obviously enjoying her company and the wine. Knowing that a Taoist will find joy and contentment in any situation, I attempted to at least pretend to be at ease, but my feet where shaking as if getting ready to jump from my stool and carry me back to the safety and solitude of my apartment.

Master Chang then spoke, more soberly than I imagined he was capable of at that moment. "Do not be so nervous. You are sitting in the presence of a true immortaless, a genuine honor for both of us. So pay close attention to what we will be discussing with you." His words jolted me out of my defensiveness. "Immortaless Chin Hua has graciously accepted my longtime pleas for her to examine you and see if you are fit for learning from her, which I have felt is best suited to you. She is the present matriarch of the sect Green Dragon, White Tigress, a group that devotes itself to the sexual yogic practices handed down through the ages through lineages from Hsi Wang Mu (Western Royal Mother). Our honored guest is in her fifty-fourth year and yet she appears as a woman in her twenties, does she not?" Not waiting for my response he continued, "Her spiritual attainments exceed many of the elder monks living here, so I am humbled by her presence, generosity, and graciousness in agreeing to this meeting.

"All your life you have suffered from weak ching affecting your kidneys and your entire physical condition. You cannot progress in your alchemical practices without first fully developing your ching. When you lived at home and you would play yin and yang harmony with your sister Mei Li, you gained a vague sense of how powerful these things can be. Our honored guest has consented to help you. I pray you accept, but it will be your choice."

A thousand questions raced through my mind. Nothing really made sense, and I did not know if I should laugh or cry. Chin Hua then reached into her jacket and handed me a note that read: "If you cannot directly face your sexuality, you will never discover your true spirituality. Your earthly spirit leads to discovering your heavenly spirit. Look at what created you to discover what will immortalize you." When I was done reading, I looked up to see her smiling compassionately at me. It was one of those smiles that can only be responded to by smiling back, and all my nervousness somehow drifted far away. The words of her note seemed to clear years of frustration and doubt, and many things I had read but misinterpreted were now clear. "Of course," I thought, "How could I miss this?" My head had been in the heavens without firm roots on the earth. No wonder I had felt so unconnected with things, like a feather floating hither and thither in the wind. Master Chang was smiling broadly at me, as though he knew my mind was clearing itself of all sorts of past debris.

Chin Hua then gazed over at Master Chang and said softly, "Good. Kindly prepare him and direct him to my household when convenient." She rose from her stool, polite gestures were exchanged, and she walked alone to the front gate and down the stone path, leaving Master Chang and me. We sat silently for a few minutes while he neatly cleaned and put away the drinking cups and the small container of peach brandy into an elaborate red lacquered box. We listened to the buzzing of the cicadas and the mating clicks of the crickets, which grew in number and volume as evening descended.

For about two hours Master Chang explained to me in detail what the Green Dragon-White Tigress practices entailed, as well as their relation to my personal experiences and interests from when I lived at home with my family. His words struck such a deep chord that tears came to my eyes. Master Chang revealed to me that my father had known Chin Hua, and if not for all his business and family concerns he would have enlisted as a Jade Dragon candidate with one of her White Tigresses. This news stunned me yet clarified why my father had possession of so many Taoist sex manuals. The abbot's final words that evening were—and I could never forget them because they rang so true for me—"Sexuality can either be a poison or a cure in a person's life, spirituality, and immortality. Chin Hua holds the cure; I suggest you partake of it."

Several days later I woke up early to make my first trek to Chin Hua's home in the city, a ten-mile or more walk from the temple. A sedan chair had been offered but I refused, thinking that for the populace and especially for the benefactors of the temple to see a young monk being toted like royalty or a rich businessman in a sedan would not look proper or frugal. After finishing my bath, meditation, and breakfast of rice gruel with pickled vegetables, I set out on foot for the city of Nanjing.

When I finally arrived at Chin Hua's front gate, tired and sticky from walking in the humid morning air, I rang the bell hung next to the door. To my surprise a huge man (Mongolian, I was to later discover) called Big Tan opened the door. Bending over to get his head under the door frame, he peered at me harshly and asked what I wanted.

Taken aback, I retreated a couple of steps and nervously said, "I . . . I . . . I'm from Heavenly Portal Temple, and I came here to see the honorable Chin Hua. She requested my visit." A big smile came over his face, which totally changed his rough demeanor. He said, "Oh, so sorry, Master Li. She has been expecting you. Please follow me to the reception room."

I stepped through the door and got a true sense of how big Tan really was. He had to be at least six and half feet tall and easily weighed 300 pounds. On his belt he held a long saber, his boots were steel-toed, and his hands were huge and looked capable of crushing rock. As we walked towards the reception room he kept apologizing for his earlier rudeness and frightening me. He really was a gentle giant, but I pitied any man who would be ignorant enough to invoke his wrath.

After delivering me to where I was to meet Chin Hua, he excused himself and went back to his station near the front gate. Her home was beautiful, lavishly decorated, and quite large from what I could tell—at least three times bigger than my former family compound. While I sat looking around at all the different constructs of her home, a young girl came with tea and politely poured me a cup. She set the teapot down with two other cups and giving me a cute smile, she scurried off. Within a few minutes Chin Hua appeared with a very surprised smile upon her face. She was accompanied by another young woman, who would have reminded me of my sister Mei Li had Mei Li been able to dress in such fine silks. She had long, black, lustrous hair fastened into a braid that fell below the back of her knees. She was obviously meticulous about hygiene. In brief, she was an exquisite beauty.

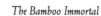

Chin Hua spoke very softly to me, saying, "You honor me by making such a long trip. I can see you walked and will offer you rest and lunch after we have a short discussion, if that meets your approval." I agreed and she continued, "I trust your illustrious teacher has had the opportunity to explain some details of what our practices entail, and by your presence I will assume that you made the decision to become a Jade Dragon." Again, I nodded politely in agreement. She then introduced the young girl to me by her initiate name, Ling I (Spirit of Ease), and informed me that Ling I had accepted me as her first Jade Dragon. We were to embark together upon the higher aspects and techniques of the teachings. I stood up and bowed low from my waist to acknowledge my honor and gratitude for her acceptance. She giggled and whispered something into Chin Hua's ear that made them both chuckle. Chin Hua explained, "She thinks you are handsome, and now understands why your Taoist name is the Bamboo Immortal, because you are thin like bamboo." I couldn't help but laugh at this myself, as I did look like a wispy stalk of bamboo, but Master Chang told me he gave me the name because I greatly enjoyed meditating while gazing at the bamboo outside my room at the temple.

At Chin Hua's home we were given quarters, an upstairs three-room apartment that consisted of a massage room where Ling I would provide massages to Green Dragons, a bedchamber, and reception room. This, however, did not come free of charge, as I was duty-bound to give both Chin Hua and Ling I a portion of the income I received yearly from the family that bought my father's business and from my monthly allocation from the temple. But all this was well within my means, and Master Chang had explained that the women of this sect needed income in order to maintain their practices, just as we at Heavenly Portal Temple did.

For three years I was to engage in the sexual yogic practices. During that time I found myself staying with Ling I more and more and returning to the temple less and less. The bedchamber was designed with a hexagonal window inlaid with glass and mica, through which I could observe and practice as she performed massage in the other room and indulged in sexual relations with other men. Afterward we would engage in one or a few of the Transformational Techniques to further our progress. Three times daily we would partake of the technique called Tigress Coils the Dragon, which on several occasions induced my experience of the Yellow Stream. I fear going into much detail of these, lest I break some vow of secrecy, but I can say that nothing within the Tao, yin, or alchemical practices I had learned previously were as potent or effective as were these experiences.

During the first six months I was given special herbal formulas that increased the size of my Jade Stem and increased the quantity of my semen. The formulas also thickened the consistency of my semen. Previously, because of all my meditation and my celibate lifestyle my Jade Stem had literally shrunk back into my body and my semen had always been clear in color and thin in

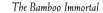

consistency; this semen deficiency was also caused by my weak kidneys. As I practiced some specialized exercises for strengthening the Jade Stem, my ching and my body gradually grew strong. Ling I once humorously commented that I came to her like a thin stalk of black bamboo, but had grown into a large thick stalk of bright yellow bamboo. My body broadened and my physique became more toned and defined. Maybe this was also a result of all my walking to and from the temple or because my increased vitality allowed me to take up swordplay at the temple. No matter the reason, it was my practices with Ling I that were the impetus for my entire transformation.

On one occasion when returning to the temple, Master Chang happened by me and without stopping he sung out, "Everyone in the world wants qi! But no one in the world understands ching! Religions all over the world reject and renounce it, except my beloved disciple the Bamboo Immortal." With a great loud laugh he continued on. I took it as a compliment, as I was sure he could visually see a difference in me and perceive my spiritual transformation as well.

One of the mainstays of the practices entailed my secretly watching Ling I massage and sexually satisfy men, usually through oral means. When this was first presented to me, I actually did not want to do it. It reminded me too much of my deviant behavior with my sister, and I really didn't see how this could possibly help me enhance my spiritual development. How wrong I was. At the repeated insistence of Ling I and advice from Chin Hua, I finally agreed to begin watching her. What eventually struck me as unique about this was that after several times there developed a detachment, a kind of numbness and indifference. In truth, it no longer felt sexual, but rather seemed like being an observer of nature. It reminded me of watching birds when I was young, an activity that would sometimes engross me. Yet because they were birds and I human, no emotional connection was made. I could become engrossed in watching Ling I and her Green Dragon, but the emotions of jealously and sexual desire had vanished. It became an interesting act of nature in that I observed but in which I did not participate.

Admittedly, at first watching Ling I and her Green Dragon was very exciting and caused a great deal of nervousness and desire within me. But by focusing on Ling I and simultaneously applying the yogic gestures Chin Hua taught me, I eventually had one of the most memorable spiritual experiences of my life. Once while Gazing at the Green Dragon, I entered a deep trance in which I could only see Ling I and her Green Dragon with my inner eye, the Original Cavity, not with my physical eyes, which had fallen shut. I was not sure if it was reality, but I had the profound sensation that I had levitated off my mat by a quarter inch or so. I also envisioned and felt as though I was surrounded by extremely fragrant lotus flower petals falling and floating around me. Ling I later said that both she and her Green Dragon were distracted by the overwhelming scent of fragrant flowers wafting through the room, and when she had finished with her Green

Dragon she entered the bedchamber to see me sitting so still it appeared as if I were a piece of dead wood. The room still smelled fragrant. I imagine I had become so absorbed in my intense gazing that I had entered a trancelike state that lasted for many hours. It had a long-lasting effect on me, as I can to this day close my eyes and with a little concentrated effort still experience these feelings.

There were two other very special spiritual experiences that occurred during my time with Ling I. The first was my experience of going into a trance, in which I could clearly see a thousand swaying lamps inside my brain. This occurred during a session of practicing the technique Soaring Dragon, Roaring Tigress. There are no words to describe the sensation; to say it was ultimate joy and contentment would not come close. Even though it felt like I had lain there enjoying the experience for a few minutes, Ling I later informed me that I had lain motionless on my right side for nearly fours hours. It was without question a life-changing experience, as even today I can induce that same experience during meditation.

The second experience was my first sensation of the Yellow Stream rushing up my spine and illuminating my brain with a great bright white light. But I must explain this further, lest readers and practitioners of these arts assume it was but a minor or simple affair. The first sensation of this simulates what a young man feels during his first ejaculation. The whole body quivers intensely, especially the spine and abdomen, with a buzzing or strong vibration that moves like a wave through the body. Every muscle freezes and is completely focused on this one sensation. When the ching and qi finally reached my brain, the tension of my whole body released, and it felt like I had been plunged into a pool of warm water and was suspended in warmth. My whole mind lit up; it was so bright yet tranquil, as if I were staring into a cloth of pure white silk.

When this state is maintained for a period of time, the body will then feel as if it is sitting on foul black tar. This will be accompanied by a loud bang or explosion, which will deafen the ears. No one else can see or hear this; it is entirely an internal experience. It is a sign that your p'o (earthly spirit) has come into harmony with your hun (heavenly spirit), releasing from your mind and body all obstacles that block your attainment of immortality. Master Chang always liked to say that this is akin to when a baby first enters the world of air and cries out to breathe; it is when our spirit penetrates and finds a new birth in the heavens.

When my three years with Ling I came to an end, my spiritual transformation had exceeded anything I ever expected. Initially I thought I might be able to feel the qi coursing through my body or grow physically stronger, both of which occurred, but which remained trivial in comparison to the spiritual experiences I mentioned previously. As human beings we can understand how physically powerful sexual energy is, but when it is used and directed inward toward spiritual experiences it becomes a hundred times more powerful.

I realize that these practices can not be undertaken by everyone; they are very demanding and took great discipline for me to maintain. Many times I felt that I had been born with great powers of mental concentration and could have transformed myself with just the self-cultivation Taoist methods of meditation, as my teacher Master Chang had done. But humans are no different from all the plants and animals of the world in that each human has its own needs for development and growth. Or as Master Chang would say, "Rice needs the sunlight to grow, a mushroom prefers darkness—each according to its nature. So it is with human beings. There is not just one path to immortality, but many—each according to its nature." For me the energy of sexuality is what was needed to pull me from my failing health and lack of spiritual progress. For others maybe it is kung fu, meditation, alchemy, herbal remedies, artistry, and so on. But for me, the Green Dragon-White Tigress practices were my salvation and transformation.

The Azure Clouds of Tranquillity Hermitage

When I returned to Heavenly Portal Temple, much had changed and so had I. The temple was in serious financial trouble, having been robbed repeatedly. Later we discovered that it was a few young novices who had figured out where the funds were kept and would fake a burglary, consequently taking off in the night with their bounty. One novice actually went into Nanjing and sat inside a box with a sign outside saying he was meditating and that benefactors should donate money. He included a small hole in the box so they could simply drop in the money. But the next morning there was no box, no monk, no money. The temple had become too popular and many came to take advantage of its wealth and reputation.

Another huge problem came during an oracle-reading arranged by a rich local businessman. A monk who was a most proficient oracle reader and medium had consented to summon the spirit of the man's dead younger brother. All went according to plan; the spirit had been summoned and the businessman was satisfied with the news and instructions given to him from his brother's spirit. However, late that night the businessman's youngest daughter had awakened everyone in the household, claiming that the oracle monk had come to her in spirit form and raped her, impregnating her with a demon child. A month later they found that she was indeed pregnant, and the rumor spread that she had been raped by the monk or a spirit he conjured for the purpose. The sad part is that the temple only performed oracles out of sympathy for the faithful. The monks living there would never even consider having it done for any of their own purposes. The truth behind the pregnancy was that the young girl had relations with a young boy, and this was just a convenient way around having to shame her entire family.

Over the next few years the temple became less and less popular, and only a few of us remained to maintain it the best we could. At one point we discovered we had been harboring gangsters who had been posing as faithful followers of the Way, but who actually needed a place to hide from the law for murdering a family in Shanghai. In order to get rid of them, we had to tell them that word arrived from Shanghai that a couple of constables were on their way to spend a week learning Taoist arts. The next day they vanished.

It was proving harder and harder to practice and find tranquillity at the temple—too many problems and not enough resources to take care of them. As the old Tang dynasty adage goes, "Too many mosquito bites to feel the itch." Master Chang and the others decided it was best to sell off the back half of the property, and he and another monk would stay to finish out their days. Master Chang hoped I would retreat to a mountain hermitage on Lung Hu Shan (Dragon Tiger Mountain) and join with a small band of Taoist masters who had completely shut themselves off from all worldly pursuits and contact. I agreed, and six months later I set off with a letter of recommendation from Master Chang to try to find my new home in a place and mountain range that I had never seen.

It proved to be a long journey, and I failed several times at locating the place called Azure Clouds of Tranquillity Hermitage. Even local residents had not heard of it, and monks at other temples along the way told me it was just an imaginary place made up by old monks to get the attention of possible benefactors. However, there was no one in the world I trusted more than Master Chang, and he claimed to have visited the place some forty years ago, as his teacher's teacher lived there. So on I trekked, having to live in the forests of this enormous mountain range, with its twisted and contorted valleys, making the terrain quite difficult when it was necessary to stray off the well-trodden pathways.

I searched what I thought was the entire area over a five month period but did not find such a hermitage, so I began to wonder if my teacher had been mistaken or if the hermitage had experienced some sort of crisis and moved elsewhere. Attempting to find my way down the mountain to procure shelter and food in the valley below, I remembered that I was not too far from the dwelling of a river fisherman that I had once come across. As I emerged from an area of thick pines I saw that I had come to the edge of a precipice. I recognized the landscape, but this was the first time I saw thick ropes tied to a tree and secured somewhere high above on top of a cliff. I wondered why these ropes were here, but as they were obviously manmade I grabbed hold of one and began climbing. As I did my body swung out along the cliff's edge. It was there that I could see a wooden platform all the way over to the left, so I swung my body hard several times until I had enough inertia to swing all the way to the platform. Once there I saw a path leading from the platform into yet another pine forest. It was but a short walk before I could see stone buildings situated within a deep half-moon–shaped conclave. I walked toward the buildings, knowing this must be the hermitage. It was so hidden, no wonder I could not find it by the map Master Chang drew. No one could see it from below, for I had been there, nor from above, as I had been there too. Nor could one see it from any side of the mountain, for I had been on both sides numerous times.

Twelve years later I left the hermitage to descended down the mountain to procure a young man in the nearest village to deliver letters to Nanjing, to Master Chang, and to my sister. I also wanted him to deliver this record to Chin Hua.

For those who might wonder, even though I am sure few remember my existence at all, my immortality has been secured. My path was long, my destiny changed, and now I sit pondering the miracle of meeting Master Chang and the immortaless Chin Hua. Without them, surely I would be in the world below, suffering and living as if drunk, aimlessly wandering as though blind. Indeed I received the peach of immortality as promised by Master Chang on that fateful day that I entered the Heavenly Portal Temple. I bow in deepest respect and gratitude.

—The Bamboo Immortal

Afterword

Organizing the materials for this book proved to be a complex endeavor because the Jade Dragon is asked to engage in several practices simultaneously, including:

1. The methods concerning the strengthening of his ching, both in the areas of the penis and semen.
2. The practice of Gazing at the Green Dragon, a voyeuristic exercise meant to develop his ching and induce ecstatic states of mind.
3. Practicing with his White Tigress the spiritual-sexual yogic positions to induce the ching to mobilize the ch'i.
4. The internal alchemy practices of meditation: Opening the Original Cavity and Reverting the Ching to the Brain (the Yellow Stream).
5. Gaining an understanding of the philosophy, practices, and goals of the White Tigress and Taoism, specifically the teachings of Master Yang Chu.

All of this, when practiced as a whole, is unquestionably a huge undertaking, and I suspect there are few men who could set aside three full years in which to bring their practice to complete fruition, as did Li Huang and other recorded Jade Dragons. Despite this, there is much in this book that can benefit any man, for all of the above can be applied in part or whole—each part is in itself a complete practice.

What is most difficult for the female in the White Tigress practices is her use of and search for Green Dragons, which for many females runs contrary to their natural bonding instincts. What is most difficult for the male in the Jade Dragon practices is his natural possessive instincts, an apprehension of sharing and watching his White Tigress with Green Dragons. An opposite instinct also exists in each, as it can also be said that most females would like to be seen as beautiful and desirable and most men are frequently engaged in looking at and fantasizing about women whom they find attractive. Underneath our socially acceptable and trained sexual behaviors, women tend to have an exhibitionist quality, while men possess voyeuristic tendencies. It is precisely these primal instincts that the teachings of both the White Tigress and Jade Dragon exploit and harness in order to achieve the benefits and goals of their practices.

Within spiritual practices we normally find beliefs about sex directed in one of three manners: celibacy, casual sex, or engaged sex. Celibacy is probably the simplest of all sexual practices, requiring only one thing, namely sustained effort to remain abstinent. But it is also the most difficult practice within which to attain internal alchemical results. And sustained celibacy can cause health problems in later life (both physical and psychological) if not directed properly. If celibacy, however, can be correctly maintained throughout one's life the effects can be very profound.

The term *casual sex* is used here to describe those who lead a spiritual life but also marry and maintain sexual relations. Such relations, however, usually lead to dissipation of sexual energy, and really have no benefit other than quelling natural sexual instincts. On the other hand, the practices outlined in this book fall into the category of engaged sex, as do those pertaining to sexual yoga and Tantra. These are the quickest and most powerful routes to achieving the internal alchemical goals. However, as with celibacy, these practices take a great deal of sustained discipline because it is very easy to get sidetracked when dealing with sexual issues. For this reason, the White Tigress practices include many rules and regulations. To be successful with any sexual yoga there must be a total commitment coupled with an equal attitude of indifference. The practices are purposely designed to take place in three-year increments, which allows the practitioners to limit their exposure to the heightened sexual energy.

Some may ask why limit the exposure? To explain, let me use an analogy that is popular in all of Taoism: The refinement of raw ore into pure steel involves both a period of heating and a period of cooling. Similarly, the Jade Dragon methods are but an effective means by which to develop ching and qi; they are not the sought after end in themselves. Sexual yogas are but a boat used to get across the river; once on the other side the boat is no longer needed. The Jade Dragon sets his mind on three life phases—sexuality, tranquillity, and immortality—each having its time and purpose. Yet there are few men who could engage in these practices fully and over the full time necessary. It is my hope that most men will at least benefit from gaining a new perspective on sexuality and women. In a society where sexuality is usually steeped in exploitation and self-ishness, I hope this work can bring some new meaning and purpose to everyone's sex lives, whether or not they are spiritually motivated.

Our health, youthfulness, and mental stability are directly related to our sexuality and sexual behaviors. It is quite sad to think that the act that brought us into this world, an activity suited to the expression of love, has been tainted with guilt, shame, and other negative emotions. Sexuality can be either a poison or a medicine, depending on the perspective or moral dictates of the individual. The White Tigress and Jade Dragon clearly perceive sex as a medicine to be taken for achieving optimal health and as a bridge linking their physical and spiritual selves.

About the Author

Hsi Lai has been a practicing Taoist for over twenty-five years, studying Chinese language, healing arts, and philosophy with many notable teachers. He lectures throughout the world on Taoism and the practices of Taoist sexual methods. He began his research into White Tigress techniques in 1986 under the guidance of one of the few living White Tigress teachers in Taipei, Taiwan.

At the request of his main Taoist teacher he went to Taiwan purposely to write and help preserve the White Tigress teachings. After twelve years of research and study he has finally finished his presentation of *The Sexual Teachings of the White Tigress: Secrets of the Female Taoist Masters* and *The Sexual Teachings of the Jade Dragon: Taoist Secrets for Male Sexual Revitalization*.

Questions about the practices contained in either book may be directed to him via e-mail through www.whitetigress.net or through the publisher.

Index

intensity of, 83
length of, 63–64
men and, 63, 79
women and, 63, 79, 86, 118
Yellow Stream and, 153, 154–55, 156

penis
anatomy of, 40–41, 61
increasing size of, 61, 62–63, 65–66
insertion techniques, 109–10, 119–20
ointments for, 64, 65–66, 81
size of, 59–60, 61, 73, 74–76, 84, 225
types of, 39, 41–49
virtuous use of, 111–12
See also glans penis
Plain Girl Classic, The. See Counsel of the Plain Girl
pleasure, 114–15, 174, 176, 189, 192
poverty, 176
praise, 192
pride, 175–76, 181–82
propriety, 187–90
prostitution, 22

qi
balancing, 132, 133, 136, 137
defined, 12, 58
developing, 14, 105, 148, 155–56, 159
sexuality and, 104–5

rain and clouds, 205
reputation, 168, 171–74, 189, 191–92, 194, 196
Returning to the Origin, 150
Reverting Ching to the Brain, 24, 25, 26–27, 147–66, 197, 227–28
revitalization of ching
about, 6–7, 57–64
exercises for, 71–86
herbs for, 64–71

saliva, 59, 94, 96, 97, 104, 110, 123
Secrets of the Jade Chamber, 105

seduction, 118–19
seeking, 168, 196
semen
color of, 30, 53, 55, 56
five types of, 51–56
quantity/quality of, 63–64, 65, 66, 69, 83–85, 113
youthfulness and, 18
sexual activity
benefits of, 5, 132–42
excess in, 59, 112, 116, 143–44
foundation of, 106–7
frequency of, 117
rules of conduct for, 101, 109–11
sensual techniques for, 108–9
seven traumas and, 132, 137–42
spirituality and, 13–14, 219–20, 221
taboos for, 143–46
Sexual Counsel of the Plain Girl, 7, 87–146
sexual desire, 99, 112, 120–27, 226
sexual energy
balancing, 101
benefits of, 229
casual sex and, 235–36
celibacy and, 58
developing, 81–82, 104–20
ebb and flow of, 113
ejaculation and, 99, 113, 114–15, 117, 208
herbs for, 64–71, 82
illness and, 57
internalizing, 26–27
positive use of, 13, 221
spirituality and, 228
of women, 120–22
See also ching
sexual positions
description and benefits of, 127–36
for Reverting Ching to the Brain, 26, 156–58, 224
Sexual Teachings of the White Tigress, The, 4, 6, 24, 149
shaving the genitals, 82
shen, 14, 58, 136, 161

spiritual practices, 13–14, 21, 102–3, 228, 229, 235
stress, 68, 113

taboos, 143–46
tan t'ien, 27, 115, 148, 156, 160, 161
Taoism, 10–11, 13, 14, 37, 167–68
Tao Shih, 215–16
Tao Te Ching, 10, 215
Three Pure Ones, 214
Three Treasures, 4, 5, 14, 26–27, 136, 160
    See also ching; qi; shen
t'ien ku cavity, 161, 162
touch, 107–9, 118–19
Transforming the True, 150
trust, 112
Tzu Kung, 176, 183

urination, 66, 145

Viagra, 70
virtues, 111–12
voyeurism, 20, 203–4, 207
    See also Gazing at the Green Dragon
wealth, 168, 176, 194
Western Royal Mother, 36, 87, 89, 92, 214

White Tigresses
    defined, 9
    Green Dragons and, 2–3, 235
    Jade Dragons and, 1–2, 18, 19, 20, 23, 236
    practice of, 4, 10, 12–13, 236
    romantic relationships and, 32
    Yang Chu and, 168
White Tigress Manual, 3, 6, 8, 64, 148, 168
women
    eight valleys within, 111
    energized by sex, 86
    erogenous areas of, 103
    frigidity in, 107–8, 133, 134
    sensuality of, 120–27
    treatment of, 14, 112

Yang Chu, 8–9, 167–96
Yellow Emperor, 10
    See also Sexual Counsel of the Plain Girl
Yellow Stream. *See* Reverting Ching to the Brain
yin and yang, 41–42, 98–103, 105, 106, 107–8, 125, 151
Yin-Yang Sexual Harmony, 98–104, 108
youthfulness, 11–12, 18, 19
yung chuan cavity, 161, 162